Plant-Based Diet

FOR DUMMIES®

A Wiley Brand

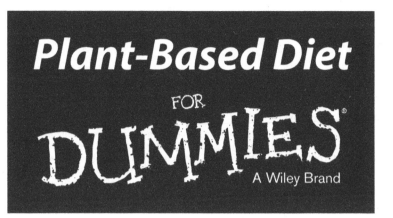

Plant-Based Diet

FOR DUMMIES®

A Wiley Brand

by Marni Wasserman

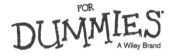

FOR DUMMIES®
A Wiley Brand

Plant-Based Diet For Dummies®

Published by
John Wiley & Sons, Inc.
111 River Street
Hoboken, NJ 07030-5774
www.wiley.com

For general information on our other products and services, please contact our Customer Care Department within the U.S. at 877-762-2974, outside the U.S. at 317-572-3993, or fax 317-572-4002. For technical support, please visit www.wiley.com/techsupport.

Wiley publishes in a variety of print and electronic formats and by print-on-demand. Some material included with standard print versions of this book may not be included in e-books or in print-on-demand. If this book refers to media such as a CD or DVD that is not included in the version you purchased, you may download this material at http://booksupport.wiley.com. For more information about Wiley products, visit www.wiley.com.

Library of Congress Control Number: 2014930402

ISBN 978-1-118-83067-3 (pbk); ISBN 978-1-118-83068-0 (ebk); ISBN 978-1-118-83070-3 (ebk)

Manufactured in the United States of America

Contents at a Glance

Recipes at a Glance

Appetizers, Snacks, and Dips

Desserts

Table of Contents

Introduction

∙∙∙

*Y*ou're intrigued about plant-based eating. You've been hearing about it, and you may be wondering, "How is this different from vegetarianism or veganism? Is this something I can do? How do I do it?" Maybe you've been thinking about how it can benefit your health. This book gives you the road map for a plant-based way of living.

Don't fret and think you have to immediately give up everything you're eating. This book uses a step-by-step approach to transitioning to a plant-based diet by gradually adding more veggies into your diet — not suddenly taking away everything you eat now. That doesn't sound all that bad, does it?

Maybe you're already mostly plant-based but are running out of ideas or don't have the resources, tools, and concepts you need to keep going. Maybe you're feeling undernourished. Whatever your reason for reading this book, I promise that you'll get countless ideas on how to get to know your fruits, veggies, whole grains, beans, nuts, and seeds a whole lot better. These foods will become your friends, not your enemies.

These foods help you succeed at any stage or age in life. Whether you're looking to stay healthy and prevent disease, going through pregnancy, raising plant-based children, wondering how to stay plant-based in your golden years, or balancing your needs as an athlete, this book gives you a comprehensive look at these phases and provides guidance on how to master them by adopting the most nutritious way of eating.

One of the biggest challenges that people face when deciding to take up a plant-based diet is mental resistance. In fact, maybe you're thinking that it's too difficult or that it's just another diet that won't last or yield the results you're looking for. Eating a plant-based diet isn't a fad or something you do just to lose weight or gain short-term results. This book is about leading a more healthful lifestyle with plants as your fuel. At the end of the day, you need to eat, so why not make your meals and snacks fibrous, delicious, and loaded with plants?

I truly believe that with the knowledge found in this book, along with a keen interest in living healthfully, you can discover that eating a plant-based diet isn't difficult and that anyone at any stage can implement a plant-based diet — even you!

About This Book

Part of leading a healthy life is setting general expectations about how you're going to approach and achieve it. This book helps you do exactly that. It provides you with the what, when, where, why, and how to start eating more plant-based foods today.

Of course, as you immerse yourself in this world and learn the basics and beyond of eating plant-based foods, you'll probably start to feel more confident. As you journey through these pages and learn about the ins and outs of eating this way, you'll discover just how easy it is.

This book gives you tools, techniques, tips, and ideas on how to fill your plate every day with plant-based foods to reach your health goals. It gives you an idea of how a plant-based diet benefits your health and what it consists of. It breaks down how much of which foods to eat and where to get your protein. It even explains how to dine out and make healthy choices in unique situations like parties and special events.

The great thing about this book is that I let you know exactly what information is vital and what's nonessential. I've packed the main body with all of the stuff I think you really need to know, but you can skip things like sidebars (text in shaded boxes). To tell you the truth, you don't have to read *anything* you don't want to read, because this book is designed to make every section accessible, regardless of whether you read anything else.

I also include some plant-based recipes that you can start incorporating into your diet as soon as you're ready. I use a few conventions in the recipes:

- ✔ All temperatures are Fahrenheit. To convert a temperature to Celsius, type "temperature conversion" into Google. A box will appear at the top of the screen; simply type the Fahrenheit number into the box labeled "Fahrenheit," and Google will display the Celsius equivalent.
- ✔ All pepper is freshly ground black pepper unless otherwise noted, and it's always optional.
- ✔ All lemon juice should be fresh and not from a bottle.
- ✔ Where water is called for, filtered water is ideal.

Foolish Assumptions

I make a few assumptions in this book about you as a reader:

- ✔ You know how to be resourceful to find new information about healthy eating.
- ✔ You're not afraid to try new plant-based foods.

- You're willing to increase your knowledge about nutrition.

- You aren't too afraid of what others think about your eating habits.

- You're eager to try new recipes.

- You want to take control of your health and are looking for a new solution that is based on lifestyle, not just diet.

Icons Used in This Book

Look for these familiar *For Dummies* icons to offer visual clues about the kinds of information you're about to read.

 This icon indicates some quick, good advice that is relevant to the topic at hand. Skimming these gives you some seriously good information that can help you implement this new diet and make your life just a little easier.

 When you change your diet and lifestyle, there's a lot of information to retain. To make sure you notice the big stuff, I call it out with this icon. Consider these the "extra-important" paragraphs you want to remember.

 Read these sections to avoid pitfalls and mistakes that could result in poor health, or ostracizing yourself or others. Learning how to eat well involves a lot of detective work to make sure you don't get tricked by confusing labels and powerful marketing. When you see this icon, it means there's something that may lead you to veer off the plant-based path — or endanger your health.

Beyond the Book

In addition to the material in the print or e-book you're reading right now, this product also comes with some access-anywhere goodies on the web. When you want some quick pointers about plant-based eating, check out the free Cheat Sheet at www.dummies.com/cheatsheet/plantbaseddiet. There you'll find a list of plant-based foods to keep on hand, suggestions for eating plant-based foods at each meal, and a pep talk about how to maintain your new lifestyle.

You can find additional information about plant-based eating in articles that supplement this book. Head to www.dummies.com/extras/plantbaseddiet for more information about using sea vegetables, starting your day with a beneficial smoothie, throwing a plant-based holiday gathering, and creating kid-friendly plant-based meals.

Where to Go from Here

Each chapter in this book is self-contained, meaning you don't have to read one chapter to understand the next one. If there's a specific word you hear or read online or in another cookbook, or a new technique you see on TV, you can use the index or table of contents as your guide and skip right to the appropriate chapter to read about it.

I've organized this book so you can jump in wherever you want, so if you want to skip to the end and read the Part of Tens first, go right ahead. There, you can find lots of good information presented in easy-to-digest nuggets.

Suppose you just want to find out about celebrating holidays while on a plant-based diet. If so, head to Chapter 16. Start with Chapter 3 if you want to learn about the macro and micro essential nutrients of a plant-based diet. If you want to cut right to the chase and try some new recipes, head to Chapters 10 through 15. If you're totally new to a plant-based way of eating, start in Part I, Chapter 1.

The easiest way to use the book, though, is just to start turning pages and reading the content. Because the true value is in how you apply this information to real life, don't be shy about making notes in the chapters, highlighting information, and putting flags on the pages.

Part I
Getting Started with a Plant-Based Diet

In this part . . .

- ✔ Discover what eating a plant-based diet means and how to start transforming your diet today.

- ✔ Find out how eating a plant-based diet can help you manage your weight, boost your energy, and aid in the fight against diseases like cancer, diabetes, and heart disease.

- ✔ Get familiar with the different nutrients in a plant-based diet, from protein, carbs, and fats to vitamins and minerals.

- ✔ Check out the new foods you'll add to your diet, including superfoods and sea vegetables.

Chapter 1

What Is a Plant-Based Diet?

In This Chapter

▶ Getting familiar with the core of a plant-based diet

▶ Understanding that this is more than a diet; it's a lifestyle

▶ Using simple ideas to start your plant-based diet today

*T*he goal of a plant-based diet is to eat more plants. Sounds simple enough — or maybe it doesn't. Eating nothing but plant-based foods is intimidating for a lot of people. Most of us are comfortable with our current way of eating and are unsure about what to do with plants: Which ones should you eat and when? Can you get full on plants alone? All kinds of questions and concerns come up, and I address some of the common questions in this chapter.

In this chapter, I also give you an overview of life on a plant-based diet. I outline what you will and won't eat. I explain how eating this way can benefit so many aspects of your life — mainly your health. At the end of the day, it's all about feeling better, looking better, and just being better, and this way of eating can do just that.

What Does Plant-Based Mean?

Eating a plant-based diet simply means eating more plants. No matter where you are, or what you eat right now, you can eat more plants (everyone can). Of course, my goal and the goal of this book is to get you to eat predominantly (and, ideally, exclusively) plant-based all the time, but you'll likely have a transitional phase, and it starts with eating more of the stuff that the Earth has so deliciously and naturally provided us.

I get to the "meat" of eating plant-based later in this chapter and explain what this really looks like on your plate on a day-to-day basis, but first I want to compare this approach to some other popular veggie-minded trends.

A few terms that are floating around represent a similar style of eating, yet they're all distinct. That doesn't mean you have to label yourself and stick with only that way of eating; these terms describe different ways of eating and help you understand what kinds of food choices fall within a certain category. Also, this breakdown can help you understand how a plant-based diet fits into the bigger picture.

- **Plant-based:** This way of eating is based on fruits, vegetables, grains, legumes, nuts, and seeds with few or no animal products. Ideally, the plant-based diet is a vegan diet with a bit of flexibility in the transitional phases, with the goal of becoming 100 percent plant-based over time.

- **Vegan:** This describes someone who doesn't eat anything that comes from an animal, be it fish, fowl, mammal, or insect. Vegans refrain not only from animal meats but also from any foods made by animals (such as dairy milk and honey). They often also abstain from purchasing, wearing, or using animal products of any kind (for example, leather).

- **Fruitarian:** This describes a vegan diet that consists mainly of fruit.

- **Raw vegan:** This is a vegan diet that is uncooked and often includes dehydrated foods.

- **Vegetarian:** This plant-based diet sometimes includes dairy and eggs.

- **Flexitarian:** This plant-based diet includes the occasional consumption of meat or fish. I like to refer to it as "a little bit of this and a little bit of that" — said with no judgment, of course!

Getting to the Root of a Plant-Based Diet

A core of foods makes up a plant-based diet. Making sure that you really understand them is key for a strong foundational knowledge that you can continuously build upon. You'll find so many wonderful foods to explore and try, but for now I introduce you to the basics and tell you what foods to avoid.

What's included

The big question is, "If I'm not eating anything from an animal, what is there to eat?" I begin by exploring the wonderful plants that I hope you get to know quite well on this journey. You'll find all sorts of diverse foods to enjoy (if you're new to this, prepare to be pleasantly surprised by what you find).

Valuable vegetables

You'll discover a whole array of veggies that you'll likely get to know quite well while eating plant-based. If you're new to this, you'll probably stick to tried-and-true, familiar veggies in the beginning because they'll feel safe — and that is A-okay! But over time, I encourage you to expand into new areas and pick up that funny-looking squash over there or try that wild, leafy bunch of something over here. You can flip ahead to Chapter 7 for an extensive list and full explanation of the vibrant world of valuable vegetables, but for now, here's my starter kit:

- ✔ Beets
- ✔ Carrots
- ✔ Kale
- ✔ Parsley, basil, and other herbs
- ✔ Spinach
- ✔ Squash
- ✔ Sweet potatoes

Fantastic fruits

Ahhh, the sweet juiciness of fresh fruit. We all love it! If you don't, you need to get on this train, because fruits are delicious; sweet; full of fiber, color, and wonderful vitamins; and so, *so* good for you. Throughout this book, I encourage you to try new ones, but here are some of my top picks to start with:

- ✔ Apples
- ✔ Avocado
- ✔ Bananas
- ✔ Blueberries
- ✔ Coconut
- ✔ Mango
- ✔ Pears
- ✔ Pineapple
- ✔ Raspberries
- ✔ Strawberries

Wonderful whole grains

Consuming good-quality whole grains is a healthy part of a plant-based diet. Don't worry; you can still have your breads and pastas, but "whole" is the key word here. You don't want refined or processed — you want the real thing. When you buy these items, make sure the grain itself is the only ingredient. Although it's possible to buy proper whole grains off the shelf in packaging, make sure you double-check the label to confirm that it is, indeed, a whole grain (and only a whole grain). Here are some of my favorites (more in Chapter 3):

- Brown rice
- Brown-rice pasta
- Quinoa
- Rolled oats
- Sprouted-grain spelt bread

Lovable legumes

Learning to love beans on a plant-based diet is key, as they're a great source of sustenance, protein, and fuel. It may take you and your body a little while to get used to them, but soon enough they'll be your friends — especially when you discover how great it is to eat them in soups, salads, burgers, and other creative mediums. Here are some of the best to start with:

- Black beans
- Chickpeas
- Kidney beans
- Lentils
- Split peas

Notable nuts and seeds

Most people love a good handful of nuts! But the thing about eating them on a plant-based diet is making sure that they're unsalted, un-oiled, and raw. As long as you enjoy them in their natural state, you can feel free to eat them in moderation alongside your other wonderful plant-based foods. Here are the best ones to start with:

- Almonds
- Cashews
- Chia seeds

- ✔ Flaxseeds
- ✔ Hempseeds
- ✔ Pumpkin seeds
- ✔ Sunflower seeds
- ✔ Walnuts

Try munching on a few nuts or seeds straight up or adding them to salads or other recipes. And if you can't decide which one you have a taste for, toss them all in a trail mix!

The extras

This is the category of foods that isn't really a category, per se, but these foods are still part of the plant-based diet. This includes such things as exotic superfoods, sea vegetables (see Chapter 4), condiments, and natural sweeteners (more on sweeteners in Chapter 13). Here are some specific examples:

- ✔ **Cacao:** The pure form of chocolate
- ✔ **Coconut oil:** Raw, virgin unprocessed oil (and the perfect butter substitute)
- ✔ **Honey:** The raw stuff, not the kind in bear-shaped plastic bottles
- ✔ **Maple syrup:** Again, the real stuff — no corn syrup here!
- ✔ **Nori:** A delicious and nutritious sea vegetable
- ✔ **Tamari:** A versatile fermented soy sauce

What's off limits

As you can imagine, all things that aren't plants are off limits; however, as I mention earlier, you may need or want a transitional period during which you wean yourself off these foods one at a time (more on that in Chapter 5) until you can avoid all things from the animal world — including meat, poultry, fish, eggs, milk, and other dairy products. In addition, because this is a clean way of living, you may cut out most processed and fried foods that don't serve your body and your health on a nutritional level.

Of course, this is the ideal — you have to find your own place on the spectrum of plant-based eating and do what works for you. Often, making something off limits just makes you want it more, so you have to strike the balance between being tough on yourself and being practical.

It's Not a Diet, It's a Lifestyle

The plant-based diet isn't the new fad or the latest thing that makes you lose a certain amount of weight in a certain amount of time. This is about changing your habits to the core. This is more than just a decision to change your food choices; it's a decision to change everything that comes with it.

How are you eating, when are you eating, and what else are you doing that can enhance, help, and sustain this lifestyle? Who else is on board with you? Do you have support? I address all these points in this book because, when you make a commitment to eat well, that commitment has to extend into all areas of your life. Eating is one of the main daily concerns we have as human beings. We need to tend to our diet in order to survive. Without food, we don't live. But also, without food there is no pleasure, no taste, and no health. A plant-based diet ensures that you get all of those needs met.

I'm excited for you to empower yourself! Any decision you make can positively impact you for the rest of your life. And as passionate as I am about that, the truth isn't in my words; it's in the results you get when you sleep better, have more energy, notice better hair and skin, and improve your vitality. Heck, you may even lose (or gain) that weight along the way.

In the following sections, I explain some of the benefits and general principles that may become part of your new lifestyle, from eating more greens to coping with your body's reaction to the additional fiber you'll consume.

Appreciating the power of greens

The earth isn't half green for no reason! We were meant to eat greens. In fact, half of your plate at mealtime and at least half of what you eat daily from the plant world should be green (see Chapter 6 for more on this).

Greens are the life force of the vegetable kingdom. Green leafy vegetables like kale, collards, Swiss chard, and spinach carry with them all the nutrients you need to thrive. They have everything from protein to trace minerals to calcium, and so much more — and guess what? They're low in calories! You can eat as many of them as you want, and they only help you get healthier. How is that for a deal? Did I forget to mention that there are ways to make them taste good, too? You don't have to chomp through them in their plain state like a horse — no! In Part III, I show you that you can get these guys into your body in myriad ways, from juices and smoothies to soups, sandwiches, salads, and more.

These powerful vegetables are the key to health. They help enliven and enrich your cells from the inside out. As long as they're kept in their prime and not overcooked (meaning, staying green and not grey or brown), they can give you all the goodness they have.

Here are the best greens to start with, from sweetest to most bitter:

- Lettuce
- Spinach
- Broccoli
- Kale
- Swiss chard
- Bok choy
- Collards
- Arugula
- Dandelion greens
- Mustard greens

And here are some ideas of where you can add greens:

- **Green juices:** Go to a store where they make fresh juices and test the waters. If you have a juicer at home, give it a go — soon, you'll be adding greens to every juice!

- **Smoothies:** Add a handful of spinach or kale to your next fruit smoothie. You won't taste them, but you still get all the beneficial nutrients.

- **Salads:** You don't have to use just lettuce. Try chopping kale and chard into bite-size pieces and adding them to your next salad. A salad allows you to get all the enzymes and nutrients greens have to offer in their raw state.

- **Sandwiches:** Dress a sandwich with any green you'd like to add a little crunch.

- **Soups and stews:** You can chop up greens and add them to your soup to give it a little texture. For those picky eaters, puree the leafy greens into a soup . . . they'll never know!

- **Stir-fries:** Slice greens really thin and sauté them with olive oil and garlic, and then drop them into different recipes or serve them alongside other dishes.

- **Pastas:** Add fresh greens at the end of the cook time for your pasta or sauce. Warm them up a bit to wilt them so they combine more easily with the pasta. (And the greens add a fun dose of color as well as nutrients.)

Try one new green a week. It's important to rotate your greens because our bodies can become too dependent on the nutrients in one and then not get others. Also, you may develop an allergy or intolerance if you eat the same one for too long.

Focusing on quality, not quantity

It's not about how much you eat; it's about *what* you eat. In fact, the amount you eat is irrelevant. I realize that may shock you, given that most diets are so focused on portion size, calories, and grams of protein. It drives me mad! Why? Because restricting food and calories is *not* the key to health. It's about what's in the food, what it's made up of, and what's in that recipe or box that counts. I want to get you so connected to your food that you become obsessed with ingredients and what's in your meals, as opposed to how much your plate weighs. You may actually start to feel lighter just knowing you can let go of that concept here and now.

Of course, I touch upon numbers, in terms of recommended serving sizes and dietary percentages, a few times throughout the book to make sure you understand approximates and to give you a guideline, but in no way do I want you to become attached to this. Instead, become attached to being healthy and figuring out how plant-based eating enriches your "nutritional wardrobe" with all the colors, textures, and features brought forth by plants.

Try focusing on eating foods in their whole forms, not out of a package. Try to introduce at least one new food a week as you transition, while at the same time eliminating processed foods.

It's all in the genes: Understanding and working with your code for health

People love to make the excuse that it's in their genes to eat a certain way, or to give in to being overweight because their parents are. Well, I say bananas!

Yes, your genes do play a significant role and help to make up who you are. But they're not the be all and end all; you can work with them and around them. You can use your genes as a template, but don't let them lock you in. Let them help you understand who you are and how you can overcome them.

You may be prone to thyroid disease, cancer, diabetes, or osteoporosis (we all are, to some extent). Instead of focusing on that, focus on how you can either prevent or reverse the disease. Flip to Chapter 20 for more on how a plant-based diet helps with specific disease prevention and control. If you have a family history of an illness or malady, take control now with your diet. You don't have to be the next victim. You can do something about it!

Forging ahead with fiber

You can never see enough commercials telling you to eat more fiber; we are a society that lacks fiber. It's from not only the processed food but also the meat and dairy that the average North American eats, all of which have no fiber. It's a pretty sad state of affairs, actually . . . so let's change that. Luckily, the plant-based diet is full of fiber; in fact, you can't get away from it! Here is why fiber is so fabulous:

- ✔ **Keeps you regular:** Fiber is the roughage from fruits and veggies. When it's in your body, your digestive system has no choice but to push the fiber and other things along and out, which makes for healthy daily deposits in your toilet bowl.

  Note: It's ideal to have a bowel movement at least once a day, but some people may not be so lucky. The goal is consistency, quantity, and ease of elimination.

Of course, it can work against you, too. If you're prone to constipation, your body may take a little longer to get used to the fiber from whole foods, so take it slow when introducing them into your diet.

- ✔ **Keeps you fuller longer:** Fiber means bulk, which means more satisfying and filling. Fibrous foods send signals to your brain telling you that you're full much sooner than foods with no fiber. Therefore, you may find that you eat less than you're used to when you eat fiber-rich foods. Also, fibrous foods require more chewing because of the roughage, so it may take you longer to chew, swallow, and digest.

Eating high-fiber foods — which take longer to eat — can mean that you ultimately eat less because your brain has more time to process the "I'm full" signal.

- ✔ **Adds more texture to your foods:** The diversity of texture that fiber offers to your plate is exceptional. Each fruit, vegetable, and whole grain has its own complexity of fiber, which adds to the diversity in your meals.

In the beginning, fiber will not be your friend. When you first introduce all the roughage, skins, seeds, and other textures of plants, your gut may have a not-so-fun time getting used to it all. Stick it out. Just eat it for a bit. You may feel gassy, bloated, and just "full" all the time, but your gut needs to get used to this and figure out how to pass these new foods along. When it starts working properly, you'll find that you depend on natural fiber from whole foods, not store-bought powders, to keep you going every day.

Because fiber draws water out of your body, drink lots of water when you eat fibrous foods to help it move along.

Common Questions and Answers about a Plant-Based Diet

As with anything new, considering a plant-based diet can bring up all sorts of questions and concerns. This book is filled with great information that most likely addresses pretty much everything that has you worried. But to nip the fretting in the bud, here are five of the most common questions about taking up a plant-based diet.

Can I get full eating only plants?

Absolutely! The wonderful thing about eating plants is that you're eating lots of fiber, and fiber makes you full! Also, the more wholesome the plants are (in other words, not processed), the more nutrients you're eating, which helps make you feel more satisfied. As the nutrients load your cells with vitamins and minerals, this helps make you feel pleasantly full, but not stuffed.

Also, the diversity of texture can help with this. Because so many plant foods require you to chew more, you actually spend more time getting through the meal. So a big bowl of salad with lots of stuff in it may not seem that heavy, but it can fill you up quite fast. I promise, after trying just a few recipes in this book, you'll be quite full!

How will I get protein?

This is always the big question. Well, I have a big answer: from so many different places! A plant-based diet has so much protein, you may not even believe it. Although it may not seem like the grams of protein add up to the amount of protein you find in meat, what you soon realize is that it's not about the quantity but rather the quality. The standard American diet provides too much protein, and this can cause many chronic illnesses. Plant-based protein sources like legumes, nuts, seeds, quinoa, tempeh, avocado, and green leafy veggies all have their own breakdown of amino acids, which build up inside your body to make a complete protein. The best part is, they absorb into your body much better than animal-based protein. You won't feel that same heaviness eating plant-based protein.

What about calcium?

What about calcium, you ask? Well, did you know that plant-based foods like sesame seeds, hempseeds, bok choy, carob, and figs are extremely rich in calcium? Almost more so than a glass of dairy milk. I know this may be hard to get your head around, but it is actually proven in most cultures that the less dairy is consumed, the more calcium is absorbed by the body.

So fret not — just because you have "grown-ups" thinking you need a glass of milk to get your daily dose of calcium, that doesn't mean the so-called experts are right. Turns out, you can eat almonds, seeds, and greens and get the same amount of calcium in your body. You won't feel bloated, either, as these sources of calcium are loaded with vitamins and minerals, making the nutrients much easier to absorb.

How do I get iron? Won't I become anemic?

Iron is definitely an area of concern for anyone not eating meat, so you need to be a bit more cautious to make sure you're consuming enough of plant-based sources such as:

- ✔ Dark leafy greens
- ✔ Seaweeds
- ✔ Nuts
- ✔ Seeds
- ✔ Legumes
- ✔ Dried fruit

If you still feel like you aren't getting enough, you may want to consider taking a good-quality, plant-based iron supplement — even just for a short period of time to boost your stores (see Chapter 9 for more on supplements).

Many people — even athletes and the like — survive and even *thrive* without meat!

Does eating plant-based help people lose weight?

I'm adamant that people should never choose to eat a specific way for weight loss. This never proves to have beneficial long-term results and always backfires on people if their weight-loss plans aren't aligned for true health reasons. Focusing solely on weight loss or calorie counting can be extremely detrimental and can take up a lot of brain power and energy.

The good news is that by following a plant-based and healthy lifestyle, you will start to feel great and lose weight naturally. When you focus on eating well-balanced and nutrient-dense meals, your body isn't deprived, and it starts to function efficiently. Deprivation is not an option.

A Quick Guide to Making Plant-Based Part of Your Everyday Life

You can start with simple ways to make eating plant-based foods easy and noninvasive to your existing diet. Here are a few suggestions to help you get started today:

- **Replace one to three meals a week with plant-based ones.** Use some of the recipes in this book (flip to Part III) or search for others that appeal to your palate.

- **Include healthy meat alternatives,** such as beans, legumes, nuts, and fermented soy, in place of meat in your meals.

- **Choose healthy alternatives to dairy,** such as rice milk, almond milk, and hempseed milk, or try avocado and cashews in place of cheese.

- **Explore new vegetables.** Go beyond your usual suspects and experiment with new colors and different green leafy vegetables.

- **Have a smoothie for breakfast.** Swap out bacon and eggs for a nutritious blended fruit smoothie to get you going in the morning.

- **Swap out butter for coconut oil.** This can be spread on toast, used in baking, and substituted anywhere else butter or margarine is used.

- **Pack power snacks.** Don't lurk around the vending machines, which are filled with non-plant-based ingredients. Bring trail mix (nuts, seeds, and dried fruit) to work or keep a small container of it handy at all times.

- **Make a simple veggie dinner at least one night a week.** If you're just getting started, change up at least one of your meat-centered meals to something plant-based yet familiar, like a vegetable stir-fry, hearty soup, or pasta.

Chapter 2

Seeing the Benefits of a Plant-Based Diet

. . . .

In This Chapter

▷ Getting an overview of a plant-based food guide

▷ Managing weight, staying energized, and sleeping well on a plant-based diet

▷ Preventing and treating diseases with plant-based foods

. . . .

*T*he plant-based diet isn't just about food; it's a framework for your well-being. Think of it as preventive health care. The money and time you invest now to better yourself through your diet pays off in leaps and bounds both sooner and later. How? So glad you asked. This chapter outlines the benefits of taking up a plant-based diet, from positive effects on sleep to weight-management and disease-fighting benefits. When you opt to transition to a plant-based diet, you make not only a positive lifestyle choice but also a smart health choice.

Eating According to a Plant-Based Food Guide

We've all seen some version of a food guide — a graphic representation of food categories divided into segments. The more space a food group takes up, the more we're supposed to eat of it to maintain a healthy diet. Many traditional food guides include meat or protein, fruit, vegetable, grain, and dairy categories. Vegetarian food guides are also available to help guide your dietary choices.

This way of grouping foods to provide a one-size-fits-all way of eating is not necessarily ideal for or relevant to everyone. My goal is to encourage you to take all food guides in stride. How much you eat and what you choose to eat need to apply directly to you and your lifestyle, activity level, and health concerns.

The guidelines in this book follow a plant-based food guide. The plan can be adjusted in cases of disease or food sensitivities, but for the most part this is an excellent foundation for superior health. Here's how this breakdown looks on a daily basis:

✔ **Fruits and vegetables**

- These should make up a majority of your overall food intake, approximately 40 percent to 60 percent, with an emphasis on leafy green veggies.

- Include at least four servings of vegetables, three of which are raw, and make sure at least one serving is green vegetables and one or more servings are starchy and colorful, such as beets, carrots, or sweet potatoes.

- Vegetables should be fresh, not canned or frozen.

  Not all frozen veggies are the same. Many frozen vegetables are even more nutritious than fresh vegetables because they are frozen at their peak ripeness, which means they maintain their nutrients. Be sure to look for organic and non-genetically modified frozen (and fresh) vegetables.

- Include sea vegetables, such as arame, nori, and dulse (see Chapter 4 for more information on sea vegetables).

- Have one to two (or more) servings of fresh fruit, preferably in season and organic.

✔ **Whole grains**

- Eat two to five servings.

- Focus on gluten-free whole grains, such as brown rice, quinoa, millet, and buckwheat.

- Choose alternatives to whole wheat as often as you can (kamut, spelt, rye, barley, and oats).

- Choose sprouted-grain products as often as you can.

✔ **Proteins**

- Have at least two servings, one of which is ½ cup of legumes, beans, tempeh, or tofu.

- If you're using plant-based protein supplements (such as hemp, pea, or brown-rice powders), use one scoop per day.

  Protein supplements aren't usually necessary to obtain adequate protein on a plant-based diet because plant protein is abundant in many sources, such as nuts, seeds, fruits, vegetables, and whole grains. Therefore, be careful not to consume excessive amounts of protein. As a culture, we are obsessed with getting enough protein; focus on quality protein and not quantity.

✔ **Fats and oils**

- Eat one serving (approximately ½ cup) of nuts or seeds.

- Have one to two tablespoons of nut or seed butters.

- Use one tablespoon of oil (grapeseed, coconut, flax, chia, hemp, or olive) for cooking or in salads.

  Do not cook with flax, hemp, or chia oil. These oils should be used only with foods that don't require heating.

- Enjoy one or more servings of whole fatty fruits, such as avocados, coconuts, and olives. This can be in the form of ¼ avocado, four olives, or ¼–½ cup fresh coconut meat.

These are just general guidelines and suggestions to help get you started with your new plant-based lifestyle. As you become accustomed to these guidelines, adapt them accordingly to what works best for you.

I'm not one to get too caught up in exact amounts or measurements of food or servings. I believe that as long as you're eating a well-rounded and balanced diet, your body gets what it needs. It's important to follow some general guidelines to get started, but in time you'll start to trust yourself because your body knows best.

Feeling Good with Food

Although it sounds simple, feeling good is really important. When you don't feel good, all other aspects of your life get out of balance — you can't be your optimal self, either personally or professionally. Luckily, you have an ace up your sleeve: proper nutrition. You have control over your diet every day, and you can choose what goes into your mouth. Choosing a plant-based diet can be extremely powerful in your quest to stay healthy. You may find that after you make the switch to this diet, you start to feel better, lose weight, have more energy, and sleep better. The following sections detail these benefits of a plant-based diet.

Weight management

Changing over from animal foods to plant foods means you consume far less saturated fat and fewer dense calories that can lead to weight gain. The calories and nutrients that come from plant-based foods do so much more for you, in terms of helping with metabolism and many functions in the body. By eating more fiber and nutrient-dense foods, you generally don't eat as much in one sitting. This may encourage you to eat more frequent meals, which is incredible for weight loss. Meat and dairy products are heavy and filled with saturated fat, and they pack on the calories. A plant-based diet is lean and efficient, preventing you from taking in food that just turns into fat.

People sometimes get hung up on the fact that following a plant-based diet means consuming more carbohydrates. That may be true, but it doesn't necessarily mean you'll gain weight. The key is to choose carbs that are high in fiber and contain lots of other nutrients. Your body will digest them well and use them for energy. You gain weight from carbs when you eat beyond your needs or you eat carbohydrates made from refined grains.

When eating a plant-based diet, be sure to choose complex carbs (such as quinoa, sweet potatoes, apples, and rolled oats) that are rich in vitamins, minerals, and protein, and enjoy them in moderation. Stay away from simple carbs (such as sugars, breads, and pastas made with refined grains). If you follow those general guidelines, you can still reach your weight goals. See more on the difference between carbohydrates in Chapter 3.

Energy and vitality

Within days of consuming more green, leafy veggies and fruits, you'll feel more energized. This is a result of the water content of these foods, which hydrates your body, providing your cells with more oxygen (as compared to meat), and it's also because of the life force running through these foods. They're filled with vitamins and minerals that infuse directly into your blood system, helping your body detoxify and rejuvenate itself. Heavy animal-based foods, such as meat and dairy, can weigh you down, decrease your energy, and make you tired. Plant-based foods are lighter and easier to digest.

Better sleep quality

When you eat better, you sleep better. I know this sounds too simple to be true, but it is. Let me paint the picture. When you nourish your body during the day with regular plant-based meals, you may find, in time, that the quality of your sleep is better. Many plant foods, such as green, leafy vegetables that are rich in magnesium and calcium, can help the body relax for a peaceful sleep. Other plant-based foods, such as whole grains, help the body produce serotonin, which has a calming effect on the body. Eating a plant-based diet doesn't necessarily mean you get more sleep — just better sleep. In fact, you may find that you need less sleep.

If you have problems sleeping, try having a banana, some oatmeal, or some almond butter on toast. These foods tend to help the body and the nervous system relax at night by causing the body to release the hormones required for a restful sleep. You can also try drinking herbal tea, such as chamomile, kava root, or valerian root, because it has a sedative effect on the body and can aid in falling asleep.

Becoming a Wellness Warrior

By committing to a plant-based diet, you become a warrior of your own wellness — a soldier defending your health. A plant-based diet can go a very long way in this fight — specifically in helping to prevent many diseases. Common diseases like cancer, diabetes, heart disease, and osteoporosis have all been known to be lessened or even reversed with a high-quality plant-based diet that is rich in fiber, phytonutrients, and protein.

The following sections explain how to prevent, minimize, or eliminate certain health conditions by following a plant-based diet. However, please be sure to talk to your doctor or health-care practitioner before making any significant dietary changes.

Cancer

Plant-based diets are effective against cancer because they're jam-packed with *phytonutrients* — the chemicals in plants that help prevent disease and infection. The more of them you eat, the better you feel, and the more you help yourself beat the odds of cancer.

If you want to prevent or fight cancer, focus on a diet that is rich in

- **Colorful fruits and vegetables,** such as blueberries, mangos, grapes, squash, tomatoes, and cucumbers
- **Green leafy vegetables,** such as kale, bok choy, collards, and Swiss chard
- **Whole grains,** such as quinoa, brown rice, millet, and amaranth
- **Legumes,** such as lentils, split peas, and mung beans
- **A variety of healthy nuts and seeds,** such as almonds, pumpkin seeds, and sunflower seeds

Diabetes

Diabetes is becoming one of the leading diseases and causes of death in North America. With fast food, sugary snacks, and soda pop at our finger-tips, it's no wonder that this blood-sugar disorder has become so prevalent. Before you inject yourself with insulin or go on medication, understand that a plant-based diet has been known to dramatically shift and even reverse type 2 diabetes. For the most part, people living with type 2 diabetes can control their disorder through their food choices.

Those living with type 1 diabetes will never eliminate their need for insulin. However, by adopting a plant-based lifestyle, they may be able to keep their insulin doses to a minimum and reduce the risk of complications.

Type 2 diabetes occurs when your pancreas doesn't produce enough insulin or your body doesn't properly use the insulin it makes. As a result, glucose (sugar) builds up in your blood instead of being used for energy.

Here is a quick rundown of plant-based foods that have special properties for maintaining a healthy blood-sugar level:

- ✔ **Avocado** contains a sugar that depresses insulin production, which makes it an excellent choice for people with *hypoglycemia* (low blood sugar). Try adding some slices of avocado to a piece of toast, blend it into a smoothie, or toss it in a salad. Guacamole is delicious too! (See Chapter 14 for a great recipe.) Ideally eat ¼ of an avocado several times per week.

- ✔ **Soybeans and other legumes,** such as kidney beans, lentils, black-eyed peas, chickpeas, and lima beans, slow the rate of absorption of carbohydrates into the bloodstream because of their high protein and fiber content. Ultimately this can reduce spikes in blood sugar. Try making a dip with different kinds of beans or tossing them into a salad. They even make great veggie burgers (see the recipe in Chapter 12). Eat at least ½ to one cup of legumes a day.

- ✔ **Onions and garlic** normalize blood-sugar regulation by decreasing the rate of insulin elimination by the liver. Onions and garlic are the base of most soups (see the recipes in Chapter 11) and stir-fries (see the recipe in Chapter 12). So consider sautéing them for your next meal. Try to consume half a clove of garlic twice a day and one onion per day.

- ✔ **Other blood-sugar-controlling foods** include berries (especially blueberries); celery; cucumbers; green, leafy vegetables; sprouts; string beans; parsley; psyllium; ground flaxseed; chia seeds; lemons; oat bran; radishes; sauerkraut; sunflower seeds; squash; and watercress. Many of these items can be combined into smoothies, breakfast cereal, or a colorful salad or grain dish.

Beyond knowing *what* foods are good to eat, knowing *how* and *when* to eat them can be vital in keeping your diabetes in check. Here are some additional tips for naturally regulating your blood-sugar levels with plants:

- ✔ Eat a balanced plant-based breakfast every day because it helps kick your metabolism into gear, which is needed for proper sugar and insulin processing.

✔ Don't go more than two hours without food. Eat six to eight small meals throughout the day. Even eating a small snack before bed may help. Eating more frequently helps keep blood-sugar levels in balance. You don't want to consume large, heavy meals because they can be hard for the body to digest. Additionally, excess food means excess calories, which can increase blood-sugar levels in the body and cause weight gain.

✔ Eat a diet high in fiber. Fiber doesn't raise blood-sugar levels, and it helps with digestion and elimination. Choose whole grains and legumes, and include large amounts of vegetables, especially dark, leafy greens; squash; green beans; sweet potatoes; tofu; and whole fresh fruits.

✔ Use natural low-glycemic sweeteners, such as brown-rice syrup, coconut sugar, and stevia — but only infrequently and in very small amounts. These sweeteners have a low impact on blood-sugar levels and don't cause them to spike as much as white sugar, which should be avoided completely.

✔ Stay away from highly fatty and fried foods because they typically contain excess processed oils, which can affect blood-sugar levels and increase caloric intake. Instead choose healthy fats, oils (avocado, coconut oil, olive oil, or other cold-pressed natural oils), raw nuts, and seeds.

✔ Remove alcohol, processed foods, sulphured dried fruits, table salt, white sugar, saturated fats, soft drinks, and white flour. Also avoid food with artificial colors and preservatives. These foods are extremely refined and have little to no nutritional value. They can contribute not only to an increase in sugar intake (of the worse kind) but also to weight gain because these are all forms of empty calories. People with diabetes should focus on foods that are rich in vitamins, minerals, and nutrients, and are beneficial to their blood-sugar levels and overall well-being.

Heart disease and hypertension

When it comes to heart health, a plant-based diet is really the only way to go. Because animal-based foods are loaded with fat and cholesterol that build up in arteries, causing high blood pressure and worse, you need to avoid them completely if you're at risk for or have heart disease. Luckily, plenty of plant-based foods can provide your heart with maximum nutrition. These foods are all from whole sources. A diet rich in these foods not only helps your heart but also promotes an overall state of optimal health and well-being. Tables 2-1, 2-2, and 2-3 outline foods that are especially beneficial for your heart.

Table 2-1   Heart-Friendly Proteins, Grains, Nuts, and Seeds

Food	Vitamins and minerals	Ways to enjoy
Black or kidney beans	B-complex vitamins, niacin, folate, magnesium, omega-3 fatty acids, calcium, and soluble fiber	Stir some beans into your next soup or salad.
Tofu and tempeh	Niacin, folate, calcium, magnesium, and potassium	Thinly slice firm tofu or tempeh and marinate for several hours before baking, grilling, or stir-frying.
Brown rice and quinoa	B-complex vitamins, fiber, niacin, and magnesium	Cook up a pot and make pilafs or soups, or top it with a colorful vegetable stir-fry.
Oats	Omega-3 fatty acids, magnesium, potassium, folate, niacin, calcium, and soluble fiber	Top hot oatmeal with fresh berries for a heart-healthy breakfast. Oatmeal and raisin cookies also make a "hearty" treat.
Almonds	Omega-3 fatty acids, vitamin E, magnesium, fiber, heart-favorable mono- and polyunsaturated fats, and phytosterols	Mix a few raw organic almonds into coconut milk yogurt, trail mix, or fruit salads.
Flaxseed (ground)	Omega-3 fatty acids, fiber, and phytoestrogens	Hide ground flaxseed in all sorts of foods — coconut yogurt parfaits, morning cereal, homemade muffins, or cookies.
Pumpkin seeds	Protein, omega-3 fatty acids, iron, zinc, phosphorus, vitamin A, calcium, and B-complex vitamins	Eat them raw in trail mixes, salads, and granola, or toast them lightly for an extra boost of flavor.
Walnuts	Omega-3 fatty acids, vitamin E, magnesium, folate, fiber, heart-favorable mono- and polyunsaturated fats, and phytosterols	Walnuts add heart power with a flavorful crunch to salads, pastas, cookies, muffins, and pancakes.

Table 2-2	Heart-Friendly Vegetables	
Food	*Vitamins and minerals*	*Ways to enjoy*
Acorn squash	Beta-carotene and lutein (carotenoids), B-complex and C vitamins, folate, calcium, magnesium, potassium, and fiber	Serve with sautéed spinach, pine nuts, or raisins.
Asparagus	Beta-carotene and lutein (carotenoids), B-complex vitamins, folate, and fiber	Grill or steam slightly, then dress with lemon.
Beets	Calcium; iron; magnesium; phosphorous; and vitamins A, B-complex, and C	Shred some raw into salad or steam and cut into slices (or hearts).
Broccoli	Beta-carotene (a carotenoid), vitamins C and E, potassium, folate, calcium, and fiber	Chop fresh broccoli and add it to store-bought soup or dip into hummus.
Carrots	Alpha-carotene (a carotenoid) and fiber	Cut into snack-sized pieces to munch on. Use in recipes such as stir-fries, salads, and soups, or sneak shredded carrots into spaghetti sauce or muffin batter.
Red bell peppers	Beta-carotene and lutein, B-complex vitamins, folate, potassium, and fiber	Grill or oven-roast until tender. Delicious in wraps, salads, and sandwiches.
Spinach	Lutein, B-complex vitamins, folate, magnesium, potassium, calcium, and fiber	Choose spinach over lettuce for nutrient-packed salads and sandwiches. Tastes great when steamed and added to cooked dishes.
Sweet potato or butternut squash	Beta-carotene; vitamins A, C, and E; and fiber	Steam in steamer basket, bake, roast in oven, or boil in a pot of soup.
Tomatoes	Beta- and alpha-carotene, lycopene, and lutein (carotenoids); vitamin C; potassium; folate; and fiber	Try fresh tomatoes on sandwiches, salads, pastas, and pizzas.

Table 2-3	Heart-Friendly Fruits	
Food	*Vitamins and minerals*	*Ways to enjoy*
Blueberries and blackberries	Beta-carotene and lutein (carotenoids), anthocyanin (a flavonoid), ellagic acid (a polyphenol), vitamin C, folate, calcium, magnesium, potassium, and fiber	Cranberries, strawberries, and raspberries are potent, too, and do well in trail mixes, muffins, and salads.
Cantaloupe	Alpha- and beta-carotene and lutein (carotenoids), B-complex and C vitamins, folate, potassium, and fiber	A fragrant, ripe cantaloupe is perfect for breakfast, lunch, or potluck dinners. Simply cut and enjoy.
Oranges	Beta-cryptoxanthin, beta- and alpha-carotene, lutein, flavones, vitamin C, potassium, folate, and fiber	Make your own orange juice with freshly squeezed organic oranges. Use the zest in marinades, chutneys, and salad dressing. You can even use it in baking.
Papaya	Beta-carotene, beta-cryptoxanthin, and lutein (carotenoids); vitamins C and E; folate; calcium; magnesium; and potassium	Mix papaya, pineapple, scallions, garlic, fresh lime juice, salt, and black pepper.
Dark chocolate	Resveratrol and cocoa phenols (flavonoids)	A square of dark cocoa is great for blood pressure, but choose varieties that have 70 percent or higher cocoa content.

Osteoporosis

Osteoporosis is the deterioration of bone mass in the body. This can happen as a result of aging, lifestyle, and diet, and many of us have grown up thinking that a glass of milk will prevent osteoporosis. Although the dairy industry wants you to believe that, the less dairy you consume, the better your bone health is! Many studies show that bone health is actually improved with a high percentage of plant-based foods (specifically dark, leafy greens and seeds) in your diet.

Top nutrients for your heart

You may know which nutrients are good for your cardiovascular health, but you may not know why they're good. Here's a quick rundown of the most commonly mentioned heart-healthy nutrients and what good they do for us.

- **Folate or folic acid** helps reduce and prevent hardening of arterial walls.

- **Omega-3 fatty acids** help strengthen heart tissue.

- **B vitamins** help reduce plaque buildup on the heart.

- **Magnesium and calcium** help regulate electrical impulses of the heart, lowering cholesterol and blood pressure.

- **Potassium** helps the heart pump and move blood through the body by pushing sodium out of the system and relaxing blood-vessel walls, thereby lowering blood pressure.

- **Vitamins A, C, and E** are antioxidants that help with overall cardiovascular health.

- **L-arginine** is an amino acid that helps rid the body of ammonia and helps release insulin. It is also used to make nitric oxide, which is a compound that helps relax blood vessels.

Dairy foods are rather acidic and can leach calcium from your bones, causing bones to break down instead of building up. Plant foods, on the other hand, are rich in calcium and magnesium and directly nourish the bones, giving them the minerals they need to thrive and help prevent breakdown.

Plant-based foods provide your body with calcium while tasting delicious. There is no need to worry about exact measurements of calcium when you're getting it from whole-food sources. Just be sure to get a variety of items in your diet on a daily basis, and you'll be loaded with the *right* kind of calcium that your body will love.

Top bone-building foods include:

- Beet greens
- Collards
- Kale
- Bok choy
- Carob
- Beans and legumes (peas and lentils)
- Sesame seeds
- Hempseeds

See Chapter 3 for more sources of calcium-rich plant-based foods.

Understanding that your calcium intake doesn't have to come from dairy may be difficult to digest, because most people believe that dairy is the only source of calcium. However, from my perspective, the foods you need to focus on are ones that are loaded with calcium naturally. These foods give your body its calcium requirements, are easy to digest, and allow your body to soak up many other beneficial minerals and nutrients.

Gastrointestinal illnesses

Plant-based eating can help with a wide variety of gastrointestinal conditions. A diet high in fiber, vitamins, and minerals can help prevent the onset and progression of these common diseases.

- **Acid reflux:** In this condition, some of the acid content of the stomach flows up into the esophagus. Eating more plants eases acid levels by decreasing or eliminating animal protein (which is more difficult to digest) from the diet. A plant-based diet also improves elimination of wastes from the body by increasing fiber intake and removing foods that may cause an increase in acid levels in the stomach. The more veggies in your diet, the less inflammation of the upper digestive tract you get because plants (especially green ones) neutralize acid levels.

- **Irritable bowel syndrome (IBS) and inflammatory bowel disease (IBD):** IBS is characterized by chronic abdominal pain, discomfort, bloating, and alteration of bowel habits. IBD is a group of inflammatory conditions of the colon and small intestine.

  Plant-based eating can be healing to the bowels. It can help stabilize blood sugar, thus promoting stable insulin levels and lowering inflammation. It allows for a more balanced intake of essential fatty acids (more omega 3s and omega 9s than omega 6s), which decrease inflammation in the body. Increased fiber in a plant-based diet improves elimination of wastes from the body, which promotes the flushing of harmful toxins. Plant-based eating is often alkalinizing (versus conventional meat, grains, dairy, and sugar, which are acid-forming), which also helps lower inflammation and creates an environment in which harmful bacteria starve and beneficial bacteria thrive.

- **Celiac disease:** Celiac disease is an autoimmune disorder of the small intestine that occurs in genetically predisposed people of all ages. It is associated with pain and discomfort in the digestive tract. Consuming plants and gluten-free grains can help someone with celiac disease prevent flare-ups, discomfort, and bloating. When you eliminate gluten from your diet, it's essential to find substitutes and alternative grains that are healing. Eliminating milk products and meat — which are inflammatory — is also critical for intestinal healing. Plant foods are also rich in enzymes that aid digestion — an extra bonus for people with celiac disease.

Other conditions that benefit from a plant-based diet

The nutrients available in plant-based foods can drastically improve your health, no matter which disease you're suffering from or trying to prevent. Plants are nature's medicine! In case you need more convincing, here are some other chronic conditions that benefit from a plant-based diet.

Autoimmune diseases

An autoimmune disease is a condition in which a person's immune system attacks itself. This class of diseases includes many different disorders that bring on a variety of symptoms. Some common autoimmune diseases include:

- ✔ **Graves' disease:** A hyperthyroid condition that causes the thyroid to enlarge to twice its size

- ✔ **Rheumatoid arthritis:** An inflammatory disorder that affects tissues, organs, and joints

- ✔ **Vitiligo:** A condition that causes skin depigmentation

- ✔ **Multiple sclerosis:** An inflammatory disease where the insulating covers of nerve cells in the brain and spinal cord are damaged

For people with autoimmune diseases, plant-based foods can help minimize symptoms, boost energy, prevent the development of other diseases, and stop the disease from progressing any further. Meat and dairy have been known to have negative effects on people living with autoimmune diseases because they can aggravate the condition, so simply removing such foods from your diet and converting to plant foods can be very helpful.

Gout

Gout is characterized by sudden, severe attacks of pain, redness, and tenderness in joints, often the joint at the base of the big toe. Obesity, unstable blood sugar, and — yes — a meat-based diet can increase the risk of developing gout. To combat it, eat fresh veggies, whole grains, nuts, seeds, and healthy fats. Plant-based eating aids blood-sugar management, helping you keep gout at bay. Because you fill up on whole foods, you have fewer cravings for and less dependence on refined grains and sugars and processed foods.

When treating gout, limit your consumption of dried beans and lentils. These items are high in purines, which can increase the levels of uric acid in the body. This is a big problem because gout results from a buildup of uric acid.

Plants benefit our planet, too

Because our planet is made up mostly of plants and the elements, the choice to eat a plant-based diet has a direct positive impact on the environment.

The resources used in the meat and dairy industries negatively affect the quality of our soil and water, the welfare of animals, and, of course, our health. A 2006 United Nations report revealed that the livestock sector accounts for the creation of 18 percent of all greenhouse gases, more than the entire transportation sector combined.

The cost of meat isn't entirely reflected by the price you pay at the checkout stand; the real price goes all the way back to how animals are handled on the land — and how the land itself is handled, including the water resources used for industrial livestock farming and in processing facilities. Then add transportation costs, packaging, and advertising, and the cost really starts adding up.

By making the choice to eat less meat and more plant-based foods, you're helping the land, the animals, and your health.

Alzheimer's disease

Glial cells, which provide support and protection for neurons in your brain and parasympathetic nervous system, are believed to help remove debris and toxins from the brain that can contribute to Alzheimer's disease. For example, accumulation of aluminum in the body has been linked with the development of Alzheimer's disease.

Many plant-based foods, especially those that are rich in antioxidants, such as green tea and dark berries, may help protect glial cells from damage. When glial cells are damaged, they lose their ability to function properly, which can affect brain function. Additionally, the increased fiber intake in a plant-based diet helps rid the body of toxins via elimination of wastes. Increased consumption of heavy-metal *chelators* (foods that help remove toxins from the body, such as cilantro, parsley, and chlorella) also helps to remove aluminum from the body.

Chapter 3

The Macro and Micro Essentials of a Plant-Based Diet

*T*he food we consume is composed of chemical compounds that are divided into two main categories: macronutrients and micronutrients. Macronutrients are the compounds we consume in the largest quantities, and they include protein, carbohydrates, and fat. Micronutrients, on the other hand, are nutrients required in small quantities to orchestrate a range of physiological functions. They include vitamins and minerals. This chapter details what they are and where to find them and even mentions some you should stay away from.

Making the Most of Macronutrients

The macronutrient category is the catch-all for protein, carbohydrates, and fats. These nutrients are the main building blocks we require from our diet to help us thrive, feel satisfied, have enough energy, and build muscle and overall health. If you're missing any one of these major categories, it can set you up for cravings, malnourishment, chronic illness, and an overall yearning to "stock up" on what your body is missing.

Sometimes people overcompensate by over-consuming a particular macronutrient when one is missing. For example, consuming a high-protein diet when you're missing carbs can be dangerous. Eating too much protein is not necessarily better; the body needs a healthy ratio of all three macronutrients to thrive and survive.

Pondering protein in the plant-based world

Protein. You eat a lot of it so you can get big muscles, right? But wait, can you only get enough protein if you eat meat? Most people think they understand protein and that it's pretty straightforward. The truth is, there's a lot more to know about this macronutrient than you may realize.

Protein is the major building block the body uses to produce things like muscle, hair, and nails and help with growth and regeneration of tissue. Not to mention, it's essential to pretty much all major functions of the body. Without it, our bodies would totally break down.

There are two types of proteins: *complete* and *incomplete*. To be considered complete, a protein must comprise all 22 amino acids, including the 8 *essential* amino acids (amino acids that your body can't produce and that you must get from your diet). I list some great plant-based complete proteins in the "Examining plant proteins" section.

It's important that you eat complete proteins; otherwise, you may experience edema; anemia; depression; poor immunity; muscle wasting; hair that is dull, loose, or falling out; low vitamin A levels; cataracts; and more.

Proteins that are low in some essential amino acids are considered incomplete. But the good news is that if you eat a variety of incomplete plant-protein foods together, they act as a complete protein — for example, brown rice and chickpeas or almond butter on toast. Even better news is that these foods don't have to be eaten in the same day — the body has an amino-acid bank that accumulates over a couple of days, after which it combines and assembles the single amino acids to make complete proteins.

Understanding what a healthy body requires

As the World Health Organization has researched this topic, it has discovered that we need less protein than we previously thought. In general, a healthy body requires at least three to four servings of plant-based protein a day. This works out to a range of about 20 to 60 grams a day. You don't have to go too crazy trying to measure everything out; the *type* and *combination* of protein you consume is far more important than the quantity.

Not all proteins are created equal! Good proteins are easier for your body to break down and absorb, while bad proteins, such as processed, synthetic, or cooked animal proteins (in which the amino acids have been broken down), are more difficult for your body to absorb. The good news is that when you eat a plant-based diet, the odds of your protein falling into the "good" category are much higher than when you eat an animal-based diet.

Examining plant proteins

Plant protein is fraught with benefits: It's relatively alkaline-forming compared to animal protein (meaning it has a nourishing effect on blood), low in fat, free of growth hormones, easy to digest, and better for the environment. And despite common misconceptions, the plant world offers plenty of sources of protein. In fact, complete plant-based proteins are found in foods like quinoas, hemp, chlorella, and soybeans. Truth be told, many plant-based proteins are pretty complete, so as long as you eat a variety of them, you get what your body requires.

Here are some sources of plant-based protein:

- **Beans:** Fresh or canned organic beans, green and yellow split peas, black beans, chickpeas, lentils, navy beans, white beans
- **Butters:** Almond, pumpkin, cashew, sunflower
- **Greens:** Chlorella, spirulina, blue-green algae, kale, chard
- **Nuts:** Almonds, cashews, walnuts, pecans, Brazil nuts, macadamia nuts
- **Protein powders:** Hemp, pea, brown rice
- **Seeds:** Tahini, sunflower, pumpkin, sesame, flax, chia, quinoa, amaranth
- **Soy:** Sprouted tofu, tempeh, edamame
- **Sprouts:** Mung bean, adzuki, pea, sunflower, lentil

Knowing protein sources to avoid

If you're committed to eating a plant-based diet, you probably won't be getting your protein from animal sources. However, you may be wondering why plant-based sources are so much better. Animal proteins (such as whey, eggs, meat, and fish) place quite a bit of stress on the body — much more than plant-based proteins — because they're highly acidic (especially red meat and dairy). It also takes much longer for your body to digest and assimilate them into usable protein.

When excess animal protein (from eating too much meat) breaks down in the digestive system, it breaks down into ammonia, which is toxic. The body protects itself by converting it into less-toxic *urea* (better known as urine) to be excreted by the kidneys. Too much urea stresses the kidneys and poisons the blood, potentially leading to kidney inflammation and failure.

Aside from naturally occurring protein found in animals and plants, protein also comes in synthetic forms, which can be damaging to your health. They're not only processed, but the protein in them has been so denatured that your body has a difficult time digesting and absorbing them.

Be sure to read labels and watch out for products containing these unnatural forms of protein:

- Whey protein powders
- Soy isolates
- Textured vegetable protein

Some particularly protein-packed plant foods include spinach, which is 51 percent protein; mushrooms, weighing in at 35 percent; beans, which are 26 percent protein; and oatmeal, which is at 16 percent.

Considering carbo-riffic plants

Carbohydrates are long chains of carbon that provide energy in a time-release fashion to ensure a steady blood-sugar level. Contrary to what many people believe, high-carbohydrate foods are *not* inherently fattening. We think that because they're made up of sugars, and refined sugars (such as fructose) in excess can make you gain weight. In reality, carbohydrates have less than half the calories found in fat. Additionally, carbohydrates have high concentrations of protein and essential vitamins and minerals, including B vitamins, vitamin E, folate, calcium, selenium, iron, magnesium, and zinc. So hooray — bring on the bread.

Research shows that women who eat carbohydrates recover more quickly from symptoms of PMS. Carbs can act as natural tranquilizers and are beneficial for people with seasonal adaptive disorder and depression.

The main function of carbohydrates is to provide a source of energy for your body. Each gram of carbohydrate provides approximately four kilocalories of energy. You need a constant supply of carbohydrates in the form of glucose for all metabolic reactions to happen properly. Complex carbs also help the amino acids in protein to be absorbed and used properly.

If you don't consume enough carbs, your body can turn to fat or protein for energy. This isn't ideal because the conversion of fat to glucose can go only so quickly and can cause a buildup of acid in the blood, creating a condition known as *ketosis*.

Comparing simple and complex carbs

It's important to understand the different kinds of carbs and how to identify them. The simple ones are the ones we want to minimize so we can focus on the complex. Have a look.

Simple carbs

There are two types of simple carbohydrates: monosaccharides and disaccharides. Monosaccharides consist of only one sugar, and examples include fructose, galactose, and glucose. Disaccharides consist of two chemically linked monosaccharides, and they come in the form of lactose, maltose, and sucrose.

Foods that contain simple carbohydrates include table sugar, products made with white flour, dairy products, whole fruit, fruit juice, jam, soda, and packaged cereals. So it's pretty obvious that simple carbohydrates should be ditched (except for the whole fruit, of course, as it contains fiber and many other wonderful nutrients).

Complex carbs

Complex carbohydrates have a higher nutritional value than simple carbohydrates because they consist of three or more sugars that are mostly rich in fiber, vitamins, and minerals. Because of their complexity, they take a little longer to digest, and they don't raise blood-sugar levels as quickly as simple carbohydrates. Complex carbohydrates act as the body's fuel, and they contribute significantly to energy production. They're important in the absorption of certain minerals and the formation of fatty acids.

Foods that contain complex carbohydrates include oats, brown rice, sweet potatoes, and legumes.

Getting enough of the right carbs

Ancient grains are some of the oldest foods on the planet. They've been used for thousands of years and are an excellent source of complex carbohydrates, which help curb appetite. These grains also contain phytochemicals, which can help lower cholesterol and prevent cancer and other diseases (more on phytochemicals in Chapter 4). When combined with legumes and vegetables, whole grains provide complete nourishment!

Here are some handy grain how-tos:

- **Consume one to two servings each day** (½ cup or one slice of bread is equivalent to one portion of grain).

- **Focus on gluten-free whole grains** (brown rice, quinoa, millet, amaranth, and buckwheat). These types of grain are much easier to digest and contain a variety of nutrients. They also cook quickly.

- **Choose alternatives to wheat** (spelt, kamut, oats, barley, and rye).

- **Choose sprouted-grain products.** (I like Ezekiel 4:9 breads and wraps because they're full of fiber and protein, are easy to eat, and make great sandwiches.)

- **Use these grains in their whole form or as ground flours,** in pastas, breads, wraps, and crackers.

Table 3-1 runs down what the different grains are and how to prepare and store them. Many of the recipes in Part III use grains mentioned here, so refer to this table if you need additional cooking tips.

Table 3-1	Ancient Grains		
Name of Grain	*Health Benefits*	*How to Use It*	*How to Store It*
Barley: A rich and chewy grain	Barley is an incredible source of soluble fiber and B vitamins. Both are essential for lowering cholesterol and protecting against heart disease.	After rinsing, add 1 part barley to 3½ parts boiling water or broth. After the liquid returns to a boil, turn down the heat, cover, and simmer for 45 minutes.	Store barley in a tightly covered glass container in a cool, dry place. You can also store it in the refrigerator.
Brown rice: A grain that's more wholesome than white rice; the unhulled and unmilled version	Brown rice is light, gluten-free, and an incredible source of long-lasting carbohydrates for energy. It's also high in fiber and contains several vitamins and minerals, as well as protein.	After rinsing brown rice, add 1 part rice to 2 parts boiling water or broth. After the liquid returns to a boil, turn down the heat, cover, and simmer for about 45 minutes.	Because brown rice still features an oil-rich germ, it's more susceptible to becoming rancid than white rice and should therefore be stored in the refrigerator. Stored in an airtight container, brown rice will keep fresh for about six months.
Kamut: A type of ancient wheat that's high in protein	Kamut has 20 percent to 40 percent more protein than wheat and is richer in several vitamins and minerals, such as calcium and selenium.	Soak 1 cup kamut overnight. Then add 3 cups water and bring to a boil, add a pinch of salt (if needed), turn the heat to low, and simmer for 40 to 45 minutes or until tender.	Store kamut in a tightly sealed glass container in a cool, dry place.

Name of Grain	Health Benefits	How to Use It	How to Store It
Oats: A category that includes oats, oat bran, and oatmeal	Oats contain fiber, which helps lower cholesterol levels. Oats are also beneficial for stabilizing blood-sugar levels and contain antioxidants, which reduce the risk of cardiovascular disease.	For all types, it's best to add oats to cold water and then simmer for 10 to 30 minutes, depending on the variety. For raw porridge, soak rolled oats overnight for a ready-to-go breakfast in the morning.	Store oatmeal in an airtight container in a cool, dry, dark place. It will keep for approximately two months.
Spelt: An ancient grain with a nutty flavor	In addition to being an amazing source of fiber and niacin, spelt is easier to digest than wheat.	After rinsing, soak spelt in water for 8 hours or overnight. Drain, rinse, and then add 3 parts water to 1 part spelt. Bring to a boil, then turn down the heat and simmer for about an hour.	Store spelt in an airtight container in a cool, dry, dark place. Keep spelt flour in the refrigerator to best preserve its nutritional value.
Rye berries: Rye berries look like wheat but are a little longer and more slender.	Rye berries help with weight loss, gallstone prevention, and diabetes management.	After rinsing them, bring ½ cup rye berries, ¼ teaspoon sea salt, and 1¾ cups water to a boil. Reduce heat, cover, and simmer for about an hour.	Store rye berries in a cool, airtight container. It will keep up to six months in the pantry or a year in the freezer.
Wheat berries	Wheat berries are an excellent source of fiber, folic acid, protein, and other nutrients.	After rinsing wheat berries, soak them overnight. For 1 cup berries, use 2 to 2½ cups water and bring to boil. Cover and let simmer for 1 to 1½ hours.	Store wheat berries in an airtight container and keep in a cool, dark place. Food-grade storage pails are a good option.

There's also a category of similar foods called *pseudo-grains*. They're actually seeds but have grain-like characteristics. Table 3-2 shows you more about the ones you should add to your plant-based diet, as well as how to cook and store them.

Table 3-2	Pseudo-Grains		
Name of Grain	*Health Benefits*	*How to Use It*	*How to Store It*
Amaranth: The seed of a plant from Central America that has a nutty flavor and can be combined well with other grains	Higher in protein than many other grains, amaranth also contains the essential amino acid lysine, which is hard to find in plant-based foods. It's a good source of calcium and iron, which are important for bone health.	Use 1 part seeds to 2½ parts water. Bring to a boil and then reduce the heat to a simmer for 20 minutes.	Keep amaranth fresh in a tight-fitting container with a lid. It's best stored in a cool, dry, dark place.
Buckwheat: A fruit seed that's related to rhubarb and sorrel, making it a suitable grain substitute for people who are sensitive to wheat or other grains that contain gluten	Buckwheat is rich in *flavonoids,* which are phytonutrients that protect against disease by extending the action of vitamin C and acting as antioxidants. It's a great source of protein, manganese, and vitamins B and E. Buckwheat helps balance and lower cholesterol levels while also protecting against heart disease.	After rinsing, add 1 part buckwheat to 2 parts boiling water or broth. After the liquid returns to a boil, turn down the heat, cover, and simmer for about 30 minutes.	Place buckwheat in an air-tight container and store it in a cool, dry place. Always store buckwheat flour in the refrigerator; keep other buckwheat products refrigerated if you live in a warm climate.

Name of Grain	Health Benefits	How to Use It	How to Store It
Millet: Millet is a varied group of small-seeded grasses, central to the diet in India, Africa, and parts of Europe. It has a corn flavor and is good for people with celiac disease or other wheat allergies.	Millet is high in iron, B-complex vitamins, and phosphorus.	Toast 1 cup of millet in a skillet over medium heat for 4 to 5 minutes to bring out nutty flavor. Add 2 cups water or broth and bring to boil. Lower heat to low, cover, and simmer for about 15 minutes. Remove from heat. Let stand for 10 minutes covered.	Store millet in an airtight container in a cool, dark place. It can be kept up to two years if stored properly.
Quinoa: A seed that has a fluffy, creamy, slightly crunchy texture and a somewhat nutty flavor when cooked	Quinoa is a complete protein, providing all eight essential amino acids. It's also high in fiber, calcium, and iron.	Add 1 part quinoa to 2 parts liquid in a saucepan. After bringing the mixture to a boil, reduce the heat to a simmer and cover. One cup of quinoa cooked this way usually takes 15 minutes to prepare.	Store quinoa in an airtight container. It will keep for a longer period of time, approximately three to six months, if you store it in the refrigerator.
Teff: A grain that appears purple, gray, red, or yellow-ish brown; the seeds range from dark red-dish brown to yellowish brown to ivory	Teff leads all the grains by a wide margin in its calcium content, with a cup of cooked teff offering 123 milligrams. It's also an excellent source of vitamin C, a nutrient not commonly found in grains. It's a source of dietary fiber that can benefit blood-sugar management, weight control, and colon health.	Cook teff for about 20 minutes, with 1 cup of teff in 3 cups of water.	Store teff seeds or flour on your shelf for up to one year in a dark, cool place, sealed in a container.

(continued)

Table 3-2 *(continued)*

Name of Grain	Health Benefits	How to Use It	How to Store It
Wild rice: An aquatic seed found mostly in the upper fresh-water lakes of Canada, Michigan, Minnesota, and Wisconsin; when cooked it has a nutty flavor	Wild rice is a source of *lysine* (an essential protein) and B vitamins. It has almost twice the protein content and almost six times the amount of folic acid as brown rice.	Put the grains into a saucepan with warm water to cover, and stir the rice around to allow any particles to float to the top. Skim off the particles and drain the water. It's best to repeat the rinsing one more time before cooking. Use 1 cup dry wild rice to 3 cups water. Cover and bring to a boil over high heat. Turn the heat down to medium-low and steam for 45 minutes to 1 hour.	Seal wild rice in a dark glass or opaque container in a cool, dark place for up to three years.

Now, grains aren't the only game in town. Other beneficial sources of complex carbohydrates include:

- ✔ **Fruits:** Organic, seasonal, low-glycemic fruits, such as apples, berries, and pears
- ✔ **Legumes:** Lentils, chickpeas, split peas, kidney beans, pinto beans, and black beans
- ✔ **Starchy vegetables:** Squash, sweet potatoes, yams, carrots, and beets

Planning meals with complex carbohydrates

Carbs are a big nutrient category and tend to be where many people get most of their calories. Because carbohydrates make up such a healthy and large part of a plant-based lifestyle, I've listed some quick ideas here for meal planning (more recipes in Part III of this book).

✔ **Breakfast**

- Porridge: Scottish or steel-cut oats soaked in water overnight and cooked in the morning on gentle heat for 5 to 10 minutes; add rice milk and some maple syrup and cinnamon (and soaked dried fruits)

- Fresh, seasonal fruit with homemade granola and coconut yogurt or cashew cream

- Whole-grain sprouted bread or rice crackers with nut butter

- Whole-grain pancakes with fresh fruit and cashew cream

✔ **Lunch or dinner**

- Spelt or rye bread or wrap with hummus, beans, raw or grilled veggies, avocado, and tempeh or tofu

- Brown rice with lentils or beans and steamed veggies

- Grain salads and pilafs (quinoa, wild rice, barley) with vinaigrette

- Baked yam or winter squash with green leafy salad, steamed veggies, and beans or tempeh

✔ **Minimal-appetite meals**

- Soaked oats or porridge with honey or coconut nectar

- Plain brown rice with olive oil and steamed veggies

- Quinoa with olive oil, flax oil, or tahini

The art of buying and storing grains

Believe it or not, there's an art to buying and storing grains. It makes sense if you think about it — after all, who goes through a whole bag of rice in one sitting? We usually use a small amount for a specific recipe, and then the rest of it sits around in the cupboard for a while, twisted up in a plastic bag. Instead, try these tips for keeping your grains great:

✔ When buying pre-packaged grains, make sure the package is tightly sealed.

✔ When buying bulk grains, shop at stores that have a high inventory turnover to ensure the freshest supply.

✔ Rather than stocking up, buy small amounts often.

✔ Look for grains that are dry, clean of debris, and fresh-smelling.

✔ Store whole grains properly to avoid spoilage (when their natural oils become rancid).

✔ Seal grains tightly to avoid attacks by insects and mold.

✔ Store grains in the refrigerator to give them a longer shelf life — up to five months.

Figuring out fiber

Everybody needs fiber to ensure a well-functioning digestive tract and to lower the risk factors of cancer, heart disease, hypertension, and diabetes. Fiber resists digestion by human enzymes, which means it reaches the colon in the same form it was eaten. This has a beneficial effect on gastrointestinal function, allowing your body to eliminate waste more thoroughly and efficiently.

Fiber comes in two main types:

✔ **Soluble fiber:** Attracts water and forms a gel, which slows down digestion. Soluble fiber delays the emptying of your stomach and makes you feel full, which helps you control weight. Slower stomach emptying may also affect blood-sugar levels and have a beneficial effect on insulin sensitivity, which may help control diabetes. Soluble fiber can also help lower LDL ("bad") blood cholesterol by interfering with the absorption of dietary cholesterol.

Sources of soluble fiber: oatmeal, oat cereal, lentils, apples, oranges, pears, oat bran, strawberries, nuts, flaxseeds, beans, dried peas, blueberries, psyllium, cucumbers, celery, and carrots

✔ **Insoluble fiber:** Increases the size and weight of feces through water absorption, increases the frequency of bowel movements, stimulates peristaltic movement, and reduces the time it takes for food to travel through the digestive tract. A diet rich in insoluble fiber is associated with decreased risk of colon and rectal cancer, decreased constipation, and a reduction in blood pressure.

Sources of insoluble fiber: whole grains, wheat bran, corn bran, seeds, nuts, barley, brown rice, zucchini, celery, broccoli, cabbage, onions, tomatoes, carrots, cucumbers, green beans, dark leafy vegetables, raisins, grapes, fruit, and root-vegetable skins

Avoiding the bad carbs

In addition to making sure you consume complex carbohydrates as part of your balanced plant-based diet, you should avoid the two really bad carbohydrates entirely: refined sugars and flours and artificial sweeteners. They not only directly impact your blood-sugar levels by triggering sharp spikes and drops but are also "empty" in terms of nutrients and extremely addicting.

Refined sugar and flour are the most processed form of carbs you can consume, and unfortunately they're everywhere. Refined sugars hide in plain sight, so you have to really be on your game! In addition to avoiding the obvious white granulated and powdered sugars, steer clear of ingredients like:

✔ High-fructose corn syrup

✔ Wheat flour

✔ Enriched flour

✔ Sugar

Artificial sweeteners are chemically made-up sugars that can work against you. They can trick your body into thinking you're getting some form of sugar, but instead they make you crave more carbohydrates. Not to mention, they're extremely toxic to your blood, liver, and nervous system. These include sucralose and aspartame, which are common in diet drinks and foods.

Eating fatty plants: Gotta love 'em, gotta have 'em

Fat gets a bad rap. We think of it as the enemy, don't we? We try to avoid it at all costs. We believe it's the source of all evil (and increasing waistlines), but here's a newsflash: We need fat. Fats are our *friends*. Or at least some of them — in moderation — are. Let's separate friend from foe.

The important ones you should know: saturated, mono, poly

Saturated, monounsaturated, and polyunsaturated fats are the three most common forms of fat that you encounter in the plant world. Fats are classified by their density and the number of carbons in a chain. Without getting too complicated, the more carbons a fat has, the more saturated it is. Here's a little breakdown, starting with the most saturated of fats:

- **Saturated fats:**
  - Don't normally go rancid, even when heated for cooking
  - Are made in our bodies from carbohydrates
  - Constitute at least 50 percent of our cell membranes, giving cells stiffness and integrity
  - Are needed for calcium to be effectively incorporated into the skeletal system
  - Protect the liver from alcohol and other toxins
  - Enhance immune function
  - Are needed for the proper use of essential fatty acids (EFAs)
  - Plant-based sources: coconut oil and palm oil

- **Monounsaturated fats:**
  - Tend to be liquid at room temperature
  - Don't go rancid easily and can be used in cooking at moderate temperatures
  - Plant-based sources: olive oil, almonds, pecans, cashews, peanuts, and avocados

✔ **Polyunsaturated fats:**

- Contain omega-3 and omega-6 fatty acids

- Are liquid even when refrigerated

- Should never be heated

- Plant-based sources: walnuts, chia, hemp, and flax

Most "politically correct" nutrition (meaning what the government wants you to eat) is based on the assumption that we should reduce and ideally eliminate our intake of fats — particularly saturated fats — from animal sources because they're to blame for things like heart disease. But don't let your plant-based diet lull you into a false sense of security. More and more, we're finding that it's not so much the saturated fats that are to blame but rather the processed food of today's modern industry and all of those trans fats hidden in most products. That means even though you're eating plant-based, you still are at risk for heart disease and other health complications if you consume too much margarine, shortening, refined oils and sugars, and processed foods in general.

Essential fats versus fats to avoid

We need to consume a number of fats on a daily basis from a wide variety of sources. The nutrition they provide is essential to your body and your health.

Essential fats

Essential fats, otherwise known as fatty acids (EFAs), are fats that our bodies need but are unable to manufacture. Therefore, we must get them from dietary sources. These fats fall into two groups, omega 3 and omega 6, which are made up of both mono- and polyunsaturated fats.

Omega-3 fatty acids are vital to the development of a child's brain and nervous system and for the maintenance and repair of the adult brain and nervous system; they're also anti-inflammatory. In the plant-based world, omega-3 EFAs are found in leafy greens, walnuts, chia seeds, and flaxseeds. Lack of omega-3 fatty acids can result in behavioral and learning disorders.

On average, you should consume one or two tablespoons of oil or seeds per day, or a few walnuts.

Omega-6 fatty acids can be helpful to many inflammatory conditions and diseases. In the plant-based world, they're readily available in avocados, grain products, nuts, seeds, and many commonly used cooking oils, such as sesame, safflower, and sunflower.

On average, you should consume ¼ avocado, ¼ cup of nuts or seeds, or one to two tablespoons of one of these cooking oils per day.

The tricky thing about EFAs is that most people get enough in their diet already, but they come from the wrong sources, such as products made with refined sugars and trans fats. This can actually be pro-inflammatory.

An overall imbalance between omega 3 and omega 6 can contribute to any of the following conditions: heart attack, stroke, cancer, obesity, insulin resistance, diabetes, asthma, arthritis, lupus, depression, schizophrenia, attention-deficit disorder, postpartum depression, Alzheimer's disease, chronic inflammatory disorders, and reduced cellular detoxification.

Your body also needs omega 9, but it's considered nonessential because your body can synthesize this fat on its own. You don't have to depend on dietary sources to obtain it. Olive oil is the most known source of omega 9, so keep it on hand at home for an extra boost — assuming that it's extra-virgin olive oil and that you use it in moderation.

Fats to avoid

The main group of fat to avoid entirely is trans fatty acids (TFAs). This is difficult because many processed foods are laden with them, but TFA consumption is linked to heart disease and elevated cholesterol levels. Also, TFA impairs lipoprotein receptors (the place where cholesterol binds) and your body's ability to process low-density cholesterol (otherwise known as LDL, or "bad" cholesterol), which eventually elevates LDL levels in the blood. This is generally considered to be unhealthy.

Not all vegetable oils are healthy!

When LDL and total cholesterol levels are elevated, many doctors tell people to restrict animal fats, butter, cheese, and eggs, which is appropriate advice. However, they suggest replacing butter with margarine — this makes the problem worse! Margarine is a vegetable-oil-based product designed to compete with butter in the marketplace. It's notorious for high levels of TFAs! Margarine is pretty much one molecule away from plastic. Do you want that in your body?

Steer clear of these bad boys:

- Commercially baked pastries, cookies, doughnuts, and cakes
- Packaged snack foods (for example, popcorn, crackers, and chips)
- Vegetable shortening
- Fried foods
- Candy bars

Watch out for hidden forms of fat like lard that are animal-based.

Healthy fat consumption

Okay, so how do you easily digest all of this information into useable practice? So glad you asked. Here's a rundown of basic tips to help you make sure you're consuming fat in a way that helps, not harms, you:

- ✔ **Choose good sources of high-quality fat,** such as olives, coconuts, seeds (especially flax), avocados, and raw organic nuts.

- ✔ **Always choose organic foods** for safe fats, as many industrial chemicals and commercial farming chemicals are fat soluble and stored in the fats of animals, fowl, fish, and plants.

- ✔ **Avoid certain fats,** such as trans fatty acids, hydrogenated or partially hydrogenated oils, vegetable oils (the high temperatures used to produce such oils destroys the nutrients in the oil), and fats from conventionally raised animals and fish.

- ✔ **If purchasing EFA supplements, contact the manufacturer to determine the carrier oil** (base oil) if it isn't listed on the label. Soy oil is commonly used because it's cheap. Horrifyingly enough, the carrier oils are often rancid upon arrival and have already drawn the antioxidant qualities out of the good oil in the capsules. (See Chapter 9 for more on supplements.)

- ✔ **Avoid eating roasted nuts** because the roasting process causes the fats and oils to go rancid, increasing free-radical damage in your body. In other words, they make you age more quickly.

- ✔ **Avoid any and all deep-fried foods** unless you prepare them yourself using coconut oil (of course, frying and deep-frying should always be kept to a minimum).

- ✔ **Always use heat-stable fats and oils, such as grapeseed and coconut oil, for cooking.** Avoid using polyunsaturated olive oil.

- ✔ **Always use pure, unrefined, organic oils for uncooked items.** Flaxseed oil, hemp oil, and olive oil are good choices.

- ✔ *Never* **eat** *any* **food from fast-food restaurants.** They use low-quality foods and fats, many of which are highly processed.

- ✔ **Parents should make a special effort to ensure that their growing children get adequate omega 3,** which is one of those essential fatty acids. It's worth it. Whatever it takes, feed your children organic food!

Meeting the Micronutrients

Micronutrients are the vitamins, minerals, and phytonutrients that help your body absorb macronutrients. A limited (or non-existent) amount of them can result in poor health. A majority of micronutrients comes from plant-based foods, so being on a plant-based diet virtually guarantees you're getting plenty! In the following sections, I explain more about the top ones you should include in your diet.

Vitamins and the plants you can find them in

The vitamins we get from plant sources are essential for growth, vitality, and health. They're the cornerstones of proper digestion, elimination, and resistance to disease. Here are some of the top ones:

- ✔ **Vitamin A:** Great for eyesight and night vision. It's found in a variety of yellow and orange fruits and vegetables, as well as leafy green vegetables.

- ✔ **B vitamins:** The family of B vitamins includes B1, B2, B3, B5, B6, B7, B9, and B12. B vitamins have many functions, which means your body needs a constant supply of them. They're helpful for managing stress, fatigue, anxiety, nervousness, and insomnia. The main food sources are the germ (the nutrient-dense component of grains) and bran of wheat and rice husks, and the outer portion of whole grains.

  - **B12:** Has an important role in aiding the nervous system and helps with energy and longevity. It's one of the few vitamins for which you need to take supplements when you're on a plant-based diet because it's not all that abundant in plant-based foods. Fermented foods such as tempeh and miso are sources, but unless you're eating those by the truckload, you probably aren't getting enough vitamin B12 naturally, so be sure to take your B12 supplement.

  - **B9 (folate or folic acid):** Essential for bodily functions and the formation of red blood cells. It's also essential for brain development and function. You can find it in green leafy vegetables in abundance — especially in spinach, kale, and beet greens.

- ✔ **Vitamin C:** Helpful to the immune system, the building of connective tissue, and adrenal support. It can be found in citrus fruits, cantaloupe, peppers, strawberries, cabbage, tomatoes, and green leafy vegetables.

- ✔ **Vitamin D:** An essential vitamin for the immune system and overall bone health. It's mostly found in animal-based foods, but fear not. This is the "sunshine vitamin," so just get a good 15 to 30 minutes of sunlight a day depending on your skin type, and that should replenish your stores of vitamin D. In the darker, colder months, you may want to consider taking a supplement.

If you get adequate sun exposure in the spring and summer, your body's reserve of vitamin D should supply your needs during the winter, so you may not need supplements.

- ✔ **Vitamin E:** An antioxidant that is helpful in protecting cells from oxidation and preventing aging and chronic disease. The best sources are grains, nuts, and seeds.

As long as you eat a well-balanced, colorful, and varied diet that is rich in plant-based foods, you should get your daily supply of these nutrients. However, in some cases additional supplementation may be required under the care of your health practitioner. As a general guideline, as long as you're eating at least two to three servings of whole grains, more than four servings of green vegetables, and two or more servings of colorful fruits each day, you should be more than on your way to meeting your vitamin doses.

Minerals and the plants you can find them in

Minerals are naturally occurring substances that come from the earth and eventually return to the earth. They're the basic building blocks of all matter! In essence, they're the life force of most foods, especially plant-based foods, that make everything else work. Without minerals, your body wouldn't thrive or function in an optimal way.

Literally thousands of minerals exist in the world, but for our purposes I discuss here only the main minerals that plant-based eaters should include in their everyday diets. In the average diet, minerals often come from animal sources, but plants can also be a source of minerals (and, in some cases, plants provide more minerals than animal sources do).

Calcium

As the most abundant mineral in the human body, calcium is the most important for good health. Calcium is known for the development and maintenance of bones and teeth. In addition, calcium is required for muscle contraction and regulation of the heartbeat. Calcium can be found in many plant-based foods, and the good news is that it is also well absorbed.

Here are some top sources of calcium in the plant world:

- ✔ **Veggies:** Beet greens, bok choy, parsley, and turnip greens
- ✔ **Fruits:** Dried apricots and dried figs
- ✔ **Nuts and seeds:** Almonds, Brazil nuts, sesame seeds, and sunflower seeds
- ✔ **Legumes:** Soybeans and tofu
- ✔ **Sweets:** Molasses and carob

Calcium supplements aren't the same as naturally occurring calcium in whole foods. Supplements may pose a risk for heart health, as they can promote the buildup of plaque in the arteries, causing restriction of blood flow to the heart. Be sure to consult a health-care or nutrition professional before taking supplements.

Iodine

Iodine is a trace mineral required for healthy metabolism and thyroid function so the body can produce and regulate hormones. The best source of plant-based iodine is sea vegetables — dulse in particular, which is also low in sodium and a good source of seasoning instead of table salt.

You can also get iodine (and other minerals) from unrefined sea salt, and in general it's lower in sodium than table salt.

Even with sea salt, you don't want to overdo it. You need so little to reap the benefits and get enough flavor out of your food! A little bit goes a long way.

Iron

Iron's found in every cell of the body, almost always combined with protein. Its main function is the formation of hemoglobin (the essential oxygen-carrying component of the red blood cell). We need iron to prevent fatigue and anemia. A variety of plant-based sources are abundant in iron:

- **Soybeans:** Add raw beans or the processed form (organic tempeh or tofu) to stir-fries, sandwiches, salads, and whole-grain dishes.
- **Dried apricots and dried figs:** Add into recipes for baked goods, granola, and trail mix, or eat them on their own.
- **Lentils and chickpeas:** You can cook all varieties into soups, dips, salads, or stews.
- **Spinach and kale:** Lightly steam them to eat as a side dish or add them into a smoothie, soup, sauce, pasta, or whole-grain dish.
- **Quinoa and millet:** Cook and make into a salad, pilaf, or breakfast cereal.

Zinc

Zinc is vital for many body functions and is part of many enzyme systems. It helps maintain healthy skin and collagen formation and aids in wound healing. Plant-based zinc sources include whole grains, such as rye and oats. Nuts and seeds, such as Brazil nuts and pumpkin seeds, are also great.

Mineral consumption: How much and how often

When it comes to minerals, make sure you're taking in four or more servings of green leafy vegetables, other colorful vegetables, and fruits each day. These are the most abundant sources of calcium and iron in a plant-based diet. For zinc and iron, focus on two or more daily servings of nuts, seeds, dried fruits, and whole grains.

Bad minerals

Yes, the mineral world contains some bad guys, too. They sometimes dress up like the good guys or hang out completely undetected. Two in particular to avoid are table salt and monosodium glutamate.

The common table salt with which most of us are familiar is a derivative of sea salt, which has, unfortunately, been processed and therefore lost many of its vital minerals (such as iodine). To make table salt, manufacturers strip sea salt and then often lace it with bleach or anti-coagulating substances to make it "marketable." Ever notice that sea salt likes to clump? Well, that's actually completely natural — the way salt is *supposed* to be. So ditch the table salt and change over to sea salt.

Kosher salt is popular, too, but it's made up of sodium chloride just like table salt (and other processed salts). It has fewer additives than table salt, but many varieties contain anti-clumping agents. I say, stay away from the kosher salt and go straight for the best — sea salt.

Monosodium glutamate (MSG) is a synthetic flavor enhancer that is traditionally used in Chinese food, but these days you can find it in many foods, such as breakfast sausages and potato chips. Understanding the pitfalls of MSG can be confusing. Regular glutamate is a naturally occurring amino acid that the body uses and needs. However, the synthetic manipulation and processing of glutamate produces a form (MSG) not found in nature. Synthetically re-creating a product of nature often produces less than desirable results. MSG has been labeled an *excitotoxin* — a chemical that is thought to have the ability to overstimulate cells to death. Many people link headaches, flushing, poor attention, and other symptoms, as well as diseases like fibromyalgia, to MSG intake.

Chapter 4

Packing an Extra Punch with Power Foods

In This Chapter

▶ Getting to know nutrient-dense specialty plant foods

▶ Discovering how to make the most out of superfoods

▶ Exploring the world of sea vegetables and how to use them

▶ Checking out phytonutrients, bioflavonoids, and antioxidants

*W*hen it comes to understanding nutrients and maximizing their potential, you'll discover more levels beyond the baseline of macro- and micronutrients (see Chapter 3). You need to consume some specific "super nutrients" on a regular basis.

Many people rely on a multivitamin or other synthetically mixed vitamins and minerals to get their daily dose of nutrients. However, plant-based foods contain so many nutrients, you don't necessarily need pills. You can eat almost everything you need to power up your nutrition naturally. In this chapter, I take you through the world of superfoods, antioxidants, sea vegetables, bioflavonoids, and phytonutrients, and I show you why and how to include them in your plant-based diet.

Enriching Your Diet with Super Nutrients

Countless research studies have shown the positive effects that super nutrients can have on your health. The beauty of plant-based foods is that they offer extra goodness that your body just loves to soak up. Some of these foods are rare, some can be found in abundance, and some even travel long distances to make it onto grocery-store shelves. So, of course, supply and demand can impact your consumption of certain superfoods, such as sea vegetables and acai, but having even a small amount of these foods and the nutrients they contain improves your health by leaps and bounds. What the Earth has to offer us in terms of nutrient-rich foods is truly amazing.

It may not be realistic or logistically possible to eat all the foods I name in this chapter. But do the best you can to get at least some — if not many — of these foods into your diet on a regular basis. They're such an important part of establishing good nutrition and upping your health game. Sometimes even just a small serving (such as a tablespoon of goji berries added to your smoothie) can make a world of difference.

These nutrients give you energy, curb cravings, and contain a multitude of vitamins and minerals. Powering up with superfoods and super nutrients takes your well-being to the next level. It's not just about being healthy; it's about maximizing your wellness potential. As you add superfoods to your normal routine, your whole being changes — for the better — in ways you never thought possible. Do what you can to work these wonders into your regular diet.

These foods can be on the pricier side because they're not as easy to come by. Help yourself out by doing some research ahead of time at health-food stores and farmers' markets before you buy so you can budget accordingly. And keep in mind the good news: A little of these power foods tends to go a long way, so your supply should last you a while!

Celebrating Superfoods

Superfoods are superior sources of essential, super-powered nutrients that our bodies can't make themselves. They are extremely nutrient dense; therefore, you don't have to consume very much to reap the benefits, such as a boosted immune system, better skin, increased energy, and much more. They are the most powerful foods on the planet and are powerhouses for the transformation to and maintenance of a healthier you. If you are what you eat, why not be super?

For recipes that use superfoods, flip to Part III and check out my recipes for Super Chia Banana Porridge, Soaked Oats with Goji Berries, Kale and Cabbage Slaw Salad, Chocolate Avocado Pudding, and Super Brazil and Goldenberry Trail Mix.

What they are and what they do

Superfoods have concentrated nutrients (protein, carbohydrates, and fats; see Chapter 3 for more about these nutrients) and provide an intense amount of nutrition in every bite. Anyone can benefit from eating more superfoods because they're so super!

Superfoods protect your body from *free-radical damage* (which contributes to the aging process), give you more energy, help your body detoxify, promote clear and bright skin, give you mental clarity, help with weight loss, and improve immunity. Some superfoods are common foods, while others are a little bit rarer.

As you venture into this new world, start out by trying some everyday superfoods and then work up to the more exotic ones. But before you run off to procure these magical treats, here's more about what you're looking for.

The superfoods you may already know

These are foods that you're most likely familiar with and are hopefully consuming on a somewhat regular basis. If not, now's your chance to get more of these items into your everyday diet:

- **Fruits:** Avocados, blackberries, blueberries, cranberries, kiwis, mangos, papayas, pomegranates, and pumpkins.
- **Veggies:** Kale, broccoli, spinach, beets, squash, and sweet potatoes.
- **Seeds and nuts:** Almonds, cashews, chia seeds, flaxseeds, hempseeds, and walnuts.
- **Pseudo grains:** Seeds that act like grains and are extremely high in protein, fiber, and low-glycemic carbohydrates. Quinoa and buckwheat are good examples.

The green superfoods

Green superfoods have the highest concentration of easily digestible nutrients, fat-burning compounds, and vitamins and minerals to protect your body. They contain a variety of beneficial substances, including proteins; protective phytochemicals (more on those later); and healthy bacteria, which help you build stronger muscles and tissues, aid your digestive system, and more effectively protect you against disease.

Green superfoods are also rich in chlorophyll, the pigment that gives plants their green essence. The molecular structure of chlorophyll is similar to human blood, so it helps build and cleanse our blood, providing our cells with more oxygen — which is just one of the reasons it's so good for us!

These green superfoods are especially generous with their healthful properties:

✔ **Chlorella,** a single-celled form of green algae.

✔ **Dark green, leafy vegetables,** such as dandelion, kale, Swiss chard, and collards.

✔ **Sea vegetables,** which I cover in more detail later in this chapter.

✔ **Spirulina,** a *cyanobacteria* (blue-green bacteria) that is a complete protein (for more on complete proteins, see Chapter 3).

✔ **Sprouts,** green living foods that come from seeds. Common varieties of sprouts come from buckwheat, quinoa, kamut (an ancient wheat that contains significantly more protein than modern wheat), sunflower seeds, and flax.

Watch out for alfalfa sprouts. Whether home grown or store bought, they tend to harbor fecal bacteria. This can make you sick — so pay attention to your sprouts.

The exotics

You may not be as familiar with these superfoods — which you may have a harder time finding, depending on your location. I include a little description of each, in case you're hearing about these for the first time.

✔ **Acai berries:** These are boosted with an array of nutrients, from B vitamins to zinc. Not to mention, they're loaded with healthy cell-promoting antioxidants. These are great in juice.

✔ **Cacao:** This is chocolate in its purest state, not heat-treated. It provides antioxidants that are superior to almost anything else in nature. High in magnesium and iron, cacao is best in raw desserts, such as avocado pudding or chocolate smoothies.

✔ **Goji berries, mulberries, and goldenberries:** These berries are full of protein and trace minerals, along with vitamin C and vitamin A, and they contain antioxidants and bioflavonoids. They also protect against chronic disease and can help reverse aging. They can be added to cereal, trail mixes, or muffins.

✔ **Lucuma:** This fruit can be used as a low-glycemic sweetener and contains many nutrients, including beta carotene, iron, zinc, vitamin B3, calcium, and protein. It has a sweet caramel flavor that is divine in smoothies, baked goods, and raw desserts.

✔ **Maca:** This plant root is used to increase energy, balance hormones, and enhance the immune system. It can be added to smoothies, cereal, or warm drinks.

Raw foods: The ultimate superfoods

Raw foods include any natural food that hasn't been heated. Technically (or scientifically) speaking, that means not above 48 degree Celsius or 120 degrees Fahrenheit. However, different experts have different theories about what constitutes raw food. Raw foods are not only loaded with enzymes (which help us break down food), but they're also bursting with all of their nutrients in their natural state. This is especially true when you choose to eat raw plant-based foods such as fruits, veggies, nuts, and seeds that are organic and local. You're basically eating food in its most nutritionally dense way. Ultimately, this makes most raw foods the superfoods of the superfoods.

Note: I believe that raw food should be an additional yet abundant part of a cooked plant-based diet. You can find so many reasons to consider this. First, depending on where you live, raw foods may not be as accessible as in other parts of the world. Second, the climate in your area may not be conducive to eating raw all the time. A warm, cooked plant-based meal is likely what you'll crave in colder climates. Last, I truly believe in variety and diversity — most people require both to feel balanced and satisfied. That's why the best compromise is to enjoy as many raw additions to your meals as possible, whether you toss them into a smoothie or add sprouts to a cooked stir-fry. The ultimate goal is to try to get as many raw foods as possible for superior health. You'll feel the difference.

Although it's beneficial to add raw foods into your life, it's not necessary to eat raw all the time. Instead, try to eat just *some* raw foods with your plant-based cooked foods. This can mean preparing a salad with a cooked meal, drinking a pure vegetable juice, or enjoying a green smoothie.

When shopping for superfoods, focus on nutrient-dense foods over low-calorie ones. Calories don't determine the amount of vitamins, minerals, enzymes, or overall nutrition in a food item. Also, look for a variety of colors, textures, flavors, and shapes. This makes your meals and snacks exciting. No one wants a boring meal that doesn't taste good!

Considering Sea Vegetables

Sea vegetables are loaded with trace minerals like iodine, magnesium, iron, calcium, and chlorophyll. They're alkaline forming, detoxifying, and an excellent addition to your diet. Whether you eat them as a snack, condiment, or meal, be sure to add some sea veggies into your diet. Sea veggies are particularly beneficial for plant-based eaters because they contain many nutrients that are typically thought to be deficient in vegan and vegetarian diets, such as vitamin B12, vitamin K, calcium, magnesium, potassium, sodium, iron, chromium, and iodine.

Sea veggies are meant to be consumed in small amounts because they're so nutritionally dense. Be careful to eat them in moderation! This may sound funny, but if you eat too much, you may feel detox-like effects, such as headaches and stomachaches. Also, it's important to be careful about sourcing your sea veggies through trusted sources. Sometimes they're preserved with other additives that aren't good for you, even in moderation.

What they are and what they do

Sea vegetables are plants from the sea (check out Figure 4-1 to see what some of these veggies look like). They not only carry an amazing array of nutrients, but they're also energetically charged, taste amazing, and come in many different forms. Most sea vegetables contain a similar array of nutrients, including iodine, vitamins C and B12, protein, iron, zinc, and many more. Many of them require rehydration before eating. Here's a little "who's who":

- ✔ **Agar:** Clear, colorless, tasteless, and often used as a natural thickening agent, it's best used to gelatinize foods such as pies, tarts, and puddings. Agar doesn't really have any nutritional value, but it's good for digestion because it's high in fiber.

- ✔ **Arame:** This sea veggie is loaded with calcium and other minerals, such as magnesium, iron, and iodine. It's subtle, soft, and stringy, and it makes a wonderful condiment for soups, salads, stir-fries, sandwiches, and wraps.

- ✔ **Bladderwrack:** This one is packed with vitamin K and mostly used medicinally as an excellent adrenal stimulant. It's commonly used by Native Americans in steam baths for arthritis, gout, and illness recovery.

- ✔ **Dulse:** Sprinkling this red/purple seaweed in your soups and salad dressings is an easy way to add vitamins and minerals to your meals. It's also the key "fishy" ingredient in mock tuna salads and Caesar dressings.

- ✔ **Irish moss:** This sea veggie is full of electrolyte minerals, such as calcium, magnesium, sodium, and potassium. Its mucilaginous compounds help you detoxify; boost your metabolism; and strengthen your hair, skin, and nails. It's also traditionally used to treat low sex drive. In non-dairy cream and smoothies, it acts as a thickener.

- ✔ **Kelp:** This brown marine plant contains vitamins A, B, D, E, and K; is a main source of vitamin C; and is rich in minerals. Kelp proteins are comparable in quality to animal proteins. Kelp contains sodium alginate (algin), an element that helps remove radioactive particles and heavy metals from the body. Keep a container of kelp flakes on the table mixed with garlic powder and sesame seeds to add extra nutrition as well as seasoning to your food.

Eating too much kelp can cause iodine overload and thyroid dysfunction, so proceed with caution.

- **Kombu:** All you need is a one-inch piece of kombu to put into your soup stock or beans. Kombu adds minerals and natural salt and helps prevent gas and bloating.

- **Kuzu:** A root starch that is similar to agar, this sea veggie is often used as a natural thickening agent. It can be used in custards, pie fillings, puddings, and sauces. It's the perfect alternative to cornstarch. Kuzu is extremely medicinal and has been used to sooth digestion because of its fiber content.

- **Laver:** With less sodium than many other sea vegetables, laver is a good source of iodine, as well as iron and vitamin B12. It has a tangy, salty taste but develops more of a nutty taste when cooked in liquid. It comes in flakes that are usually purplish. When hydrated, the flakes can hold about four times their dry weight. Most often, laver flakes are used in stir-fries, seafood chowders, and dips. They can also be used in salads or salad dressings for flavor.

- **Nori:** This is one of the most widely known sea vegetables. Most people have it in sushi, but it can also be eaten as a snack or added to miso soup. Nori contains vitamins A, B, C, and E and has chlorophyll and a wide spectrum of minerals.

- **Sea palm:** American arame grows only on the Pacific coast of North America. One of my favorites, it has a sweet, salty taste that goes especially well as a vegetable, rice, or salad topping.

- **Wakame:** Full of magnesium, iodine, calcium, and iron, wakame has a subtly sweet flavor and is often used in soups and salads.

The skinny on sea vegetables

Sea vegetables have been hotly debated recently because of their potential to be contaminated with heavy metals from the waters in which they grow. Although sea vegetables are rich sources of minerals, calcium, iron, and iodine, they can also act like a sponge and soak up unwanted contaminants. Arsenic is most problematic in types such as hijiki, kombu, and nori, but hijiki seems to be the most risky.

Although most people don't eat sea vegetables in quantities that can pose risk, it's still good to be aware. Also, most problems can be avoided if you make a conscious effort to purchase certified organic varieties of dried seaweeds that can be reconstituted at home.

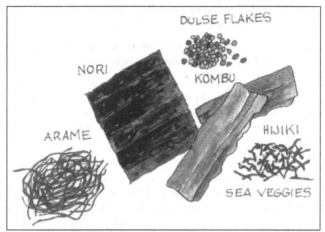

Figure 4-1:
Keeping a few different sea veggies on hand at all times makes it easy to incorporate them into your meals.

Having trouble finding these items? Try hitting up Asian markets, where these foods are more common. Don't be afraid to ask a friend to come along for help if needed!

How to use them

When you know what sea veggies are and how to eat them, the next question is this: How the heck do you cook them to make the most of their nutrients? The following tips on preparation and cooking techniques can help you make sure to get them right.

Preparation quick tips

Use these quick how-tos to get your sea veggies ready.

- ✔ **Dulse:** You can usually add dulse to your recipe without soaking it first. Just rinse it quickly under cool running water. Using a rocking motion with your chef's knife, chop it to the desired size.

- ✔ **Arame:** Place it in a small strainer and rinse. Then place it in a bowl of warm water and soak for about 20 minutes. Strain and rinse again. Chop it to the desired size.

- ✔ **Kombu:** Rinse it first under running water for a short time and then place it in warm water until it's soft. Kombu usually takes 10 to 15 minutes to soften. Chop it and add it to your recipe.

- ✔ **Wakame:** Rinse your wakame under cool running water for a short time and then soak it in a bowl of warm water. Wakame softens fairly quickly, in five to seven minutes. Chop it and add it to your recipe.

Book an appointment at the sea veggie spa!

If your stomach flips at the thought of actually eating a sea vegetable, don't fret — there's still hope for you. It turns out, there's more than one way to ingest a sea veggie.

You don't have to actually *eat* these green gems to get their nutritional benefit. It's true! It's easy for your skin to absorb sea veggies' nutrients — and your skin becomes very happy when it gets to soak up those minerals. Many kinds of seaweed are used in all sorts of spa treatments, such as foot baths, body wraps, facial scrubs, and cleansers. The richness and density of the minerals are detoxifying and

regenerative for your skin and organs. Look up local spas to inquire about their special treatments.

If you can't make it to a spa, you can make your own concoctions at home. Just soak some wakame or any other sea veggie in water, then remove the veggies and add the water to your next bath, or rinse your face with it as a toner. You're likely to feel and see differences right away. As for the soaked veggies, you can apply them to your feet or face for your own seaweed wraps. They're very nourishing to the skin.

Healthy cooking for sea vegetables

Try these easy ways to cook some of these mysterious-sounding foods. Not so mysterious anymore, huh?

- **Kombu:** Add chopped kombu to soup and simmer for at least ten minutes before adding any other sea vegetables, as kombu takes longer to cook. Cook for at least 20 minutes.

- **Wakame:** Wakame softens quickly and takes very little time to cook. Chop it and add it to soup, and then cook it for only five to ten minutes.

- **Nori:** You can usually buy nori already toasted. If it's not, you can toast it in a 350-degree oven for one to two minutes, until the nori changes color from dark purple-black to phosphorescent green. My preference, however, is to use raw nori to keep all the nutrients intact.

The water you use to soak sea vegetables becomes very nutritious and flavorful and can be used in the recipe you're making. To gain maximum flavor and nutrition, use no more water to soak your sea vegetables than can be incorporated into the recipe.

Favoring Phytonutrients

Phytonutrients (or phytochemicals) are the major contributors to the color, taste, and smell of many plant-based foods. The word is also an umbrella term for the compounds that plants make that improve a human's health. These gems possess natural chemicals that protect plants from germs, fungi, bugs, and other unsavory characters. This brilliance gives us a glimpse of what they can do in our bodies, as well, in terms of overall wellness. For more about the specifics, read on.

What they do

Phytonutrients are small compounds that have powerful results. Knowing the different subcategories, such as tannins, flavonoids, and alkaloids, may not be as useful as understanding what phytonutrients do. Here are just some of the wonderful benefits they offer:

- ✔ Antioxidant
- ✔ Antibiotic
- ✔ Cancer preventive
- ✔ Anti-inflammatory
- ✔ Tissue supportive
- ✔ Immune supportive
- ✔ Tissue protective

You can read more about these benefits in the pages ahead.

Where to find them

Phytonutrients are pretty much everywhere in plant land, which means you probably don't have to go out of your way to buy unfamiliar foods. They exist most prolifically in:

- ✔ Beans
- ✔ Fruits, vegetables, and herbs
- ✔ Nuts and seeds
- ✔ Tea
- ✔ Whole grains

Biting into Bioflavonoids

Although phytonutrients come in many forms, *bioflavonoids* (sometimes they're just called *flavonoids*) are extra important because they're among the most powerful.

What they are and what they do

Bioflavonoids are plant pigments that give color to many fruits and flowers, and they're sometimes referred to as "vitamin P." They're the water-soluble companion to ascorbic acid (a form of vitamin C). As a result, they're easily absorbed through the intestines. Although some are stored in the body, most excess is eliminated via perspiration and urine.

Flavonoids act as antioxidants, antibiotics, anti-inflammatories, and even cancer preventives. Another wonderful benefit is that they maintain the health of collagen, a protein that strengthens and protects various bodily structures (such as skin, smooth muscle, blood vessels, organs, hair, nails, bone, and cartilage).

Where to find them

Because flavonoids are so foundational to plant life, they're easily available. You needn't make any special trips to special stores; you only need to make sure you have a nice supply of fresh fruits and veggies at all times. Here's a little list of the more flavonoid-laden foods to get you started:

- ✔ Apricots
- ✔ Blackberries
- ✔ Black currants
- ✔ Broccoli
- ✔ Buckwheat
- ✔ Cherries
- ✔ Citrus fruits
- ✔ Dark chocolate
- ✔ Grapes
- ✔ Green bell peppers
- ✔ Papayas
- ✔ Rose hips
- ✔ Tomatoes

Acknowledging Antioxidants

When you're on a plant-based diet, you naturally consume large quantities of antioxidants without having to think about it too much. However, they're very important and helpful little guys, so I want to go into a bit more detail so you know why they're so cool — and which foods contain them.

What they are and what they do

Antioxidants are protective compounds that prevent cells and tissues from being damaged by clearing your system of *free radicals*. No, they aren't some sort of rogue punk rockers; free radicals are chemically unstable oxygen atoms that have one or more unpaired electrons. They steal electrons from other atoms in your body, which can cause damage to your cells, proteins, and DNA.

Because of their ability to shoo away the bad guys, antioxidants have also been known to help in the fight against several degenerative and age-related diseases, such as:

- Alzheimer's disease
- Cancer
- Cardiovascular disease
- Cataracts and macular degeneration
- Cognitive impairment

Where to find them

Antioxidants are everywhere! Here are some favorites:

- **Fruits:** Berries (strawberries, blueberries, acai berries, goji berries), plums, pomegranates, grapes, pumpkin, mangoes, apricots, tomatoes, and apples
- **Veggies:** Broccoli, cabbage, cauliflower, kale, eggplant, carrots, spinach, and red bell peppers
- **Roots and shoots:** Green tea, parsley, garlic, leeks, and onions
- **Legumes:** Black beans, pinto beans, kidney beans

Getting antioxidants another way: Fruity facials

Your skin loves to soak in the antioxidants in fruits and veggies. It's true! Many spas use extracts of these foods for creams, cleansers, exfoliates, and the like, so look for products that are made from some of the foods I discuss in this chapter. For example, excellent toners are made from acids such as lemon juice and apple-cider vinegar. You can even just dab some steeped green tea on your face to prevent wrinkling.

And you know what the best part is? You can do this at home! Do some Internet research to find cool ideas or try this antioxidant-rich Scrumptious Strawberry Mask recipe to get you started. (I dare you not to eat it.) It's super easy:

1. Start with ½ cup mashed fresh strawberries.

2. Add 1 tablespoon Manuka honey. (Manuka honey is from New Zealand and is one of the most medicinal honeys to use topically on the skin.)

3. Mix together in a bowl and apply directly to your face, chunks and all. If some gets into your mouth, it will taste great! Leave it on for at least 15 minutes to get the benefits.

4. To make this mask into an exfoliation scrub, add 2 tablespoons of almond meal or ground almonds.

It kind of makes you look like an Oompa-Loompa for a minute, but who cares?

Chocolate is the ultimate antioxidant! Because chocolate is a bean, it counts as an antioxidant — in fact, one of the most concentrated sources of antioxidants, especially in the pure, raw, and natural form known as cacao. So be sure to get your daily dose. Yes, you heard me, daily if you want. Whether it's a tablespoon of pure cacao powder or a square (or two) of dairy-free dark chocolate, go for it!

Part II
Embracing Plant-Based Living

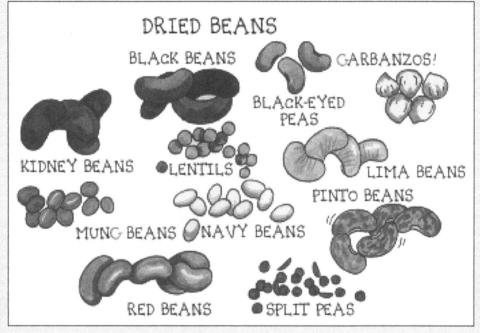

Illustration by Elizabeth Kurtzman

As part of your new diet, you'll be eating some foods you're probably unfamiliar with. In an article at www.dummies.com/extras/plantbaseddiet, I give you a list of foods that work well with sea vegetables.

In this part . . .

✔ Get the details on how to move from your current dietary habits to a plant-based diet.

✔ Explore the foods you can dish up on your plant-based plate and check out some ideas for different meal plans.

✔ Fill your kitchen with plant-based foods and figure out what equipment you may need.

✔ Know where to shop and what to look for when it's time to restock your cupboard shelves.

✔ Figure out which supplements are necessary on a plant-based diet.

Chapter 5

Taking the Plunge into a Plant-Based Diet

In This Chapter

▶ Choosing between an immediate transition and a gradual shift

▶ Finding some folks to lean on

▶ Facing and overcoming common challenges

*R*eady to make the move and become a full-fledged "plant-a-tarian"? Well, you're in good company — many people take the plunge every day to join the millions who already enjoy this diet. If you want to move forward with implementing a plant-based diet, the first goal is to understand your reasons for doing so and to choose a transition method that makes sense and is easy for you. Of course, a big transition may present some unexpected challenges (as with anything new), but it's possible to set yourself up to enjoy the process.

In this chapter, I outline how to approach your transition to a plant-based lifestyle so it works best for you. Additionally, I explain some common obstacles and ways to overcome them. In no time at all, you'll be ready to take on this new diet with gusto!

Transitioning to a Plant-Based Diet

Getting started on a plant-based diet can seem a little daunting at first, but the good news is that you can do it relatively easily and at your own pace. Whether you change your lifestyle overnight or over the course of months or years, the main thing is to prepare yourself mentally and physically for the big changes you're going to experience.

A key part of preparing yourself is remaining mindful that this is more than just a dietary change; it's also a lifestyle change, so it's normal to feel a little overwhelmed or nervous. And you should expect that a shift like this may be difficult at times. Perhaps you're working through this transition because you want to lead a more ethical or environmentally friendly life. Or maybe you want to improve your health or the health of your family. Whatever your personal reasons and goals, keeping those thoughts in the front of your mind can help you stay focused and motivated during the tougher moments.

 Your body and mind reap the benefits of a plant-based diet almost immediately, regardless of how you approach the transition. Sometimes getting started can be the scariest part of a new experience, but remembering that you'll see progress quickly can help you take the leap.

In this section, I help you figure out which way works best for you, whether it's jumping into the deep end or slowly getting your feet wet.

 To add some extra fun, encourage your friends and family to participate and support the well-known Meatless Mondays campaign (do a web search for more info) or make up your own variation like Turnip Tuesdays (well, maybe not, but you get the idea).

Going cold turkey

Removing all meat, poultry, fish, dairy, and eggs at once can feel like a dramatic change, but on the other hand this method keeps things pretty simple — no fuss, no muss. Some people, when they make a decision, need to hurry up and implement it before they change their minds. Going cold turkey has its benefits and drawbacks.

Benefits to going all in

Switching 100 percent to a plant-based diet can pay off for your body, mind, and spirit. Check out these advantages:

- ✔ When you go cold turkey, improvements in your health and overall well-being generally appear quickly. Your body is likely to respond well to eating more fiber- and nutrient-rich foods.

- ✔ Switching over immediately creates a dramatic example for your friends and family to see. It not only makes you publicly accountable (if you're the sort who thrives on external motivation), but your level of commitment may even inspire others to take on a plant-based diet, which means you may have company. Extra bonus: If you're making the switch for animal-rights or environmental reasons, your example can set off a positive chain reaction.

✔ This method gives you something to fully focus on and keeps your mind (and body) busy with what to eat next, what you need to buy, and what you need to figure out about nutrition. Going cold turkey gives you the opportunity to really "sink your teeth" into something!

Drawbacks to the quick switch

When you make a sudden change, you may experience unexpected consequences. In most cases, you can overcome the drawbacks if you just give yourself some time to adjust. Here are some drawbacks to suddenly converting your diet to a plant-based approach:

✔ Your body may not match your mind — you may have made the decision to change your lifestyle, but your body may not be ready for it. Often when you drastically change your diet, you begin to detox. This may sound good in theory, but it doesn't feel so good when you're experiencing constant headaches, bloating, and discomfort, so be sure to consult your doctor or naturopath about whether this method is appropriate for you (more on this later in the chapter).

✔ Your wallet takes a beating. Not only is replacing your kitchen inventory a significant cost, but it may end up costing extra because you aren't used to your new food-purchasing patterns. You may aimlessly try to fill in the blanks of your new meals without knowing quite what to buy, which may lead to some expensive mistakes.

✔ When you jump into something too fast, you may not really understand what you're doing and why you're doing it. You may be eating foods that aren't even that healthy or in line with your new philosophy because you haven't done your research yet.

Sometimes taking a big staple out of your diet abruptly can make it more likely that you'll get off track. Before you try the cold-turkey approach, make sure that you have enough resources to get you started so you don't feel overwhelmed.

Steps to making the switch

After you've decided to eliminate all foods that aren't plant-based from your diet, you need to have a couple of conversations with near and dear friends and family. Then you need to take some strategic steps to ensure that you maintain your new lifestyle and realize some success quickly.

✔ Tell your family or housemates about your plan and discuss whether the whole household will be going plant-based. If so, set some time aside to clean out your fridge, pantry, and cabinets together. (Think about donating those items to your local food bank.) If not, talk about distinguishing certain areas of your kitchen or certain pots and pans as "plant-based," if needed.

✔ If you're not sure whether something you have in your kitchen is entirely plant-based, read the labels and "added ingredients" thoroughly. If you're still not sure, search online for unknown ingredients.

✔ Talk to your doctor or naturopath about any health concerns you may have and how to go about the transition properly.

✔ Go shopping for new plant-based goodies to fill your fridge and pantry back up (see my suggested shopping list in Chapter 6).

✔ For your first plant-based meal, plan something easy or go out to eat. Don't put added pressure on yourself to make an extravagant meal.

Going plant-based gradually

Some people prefer the softer approach of easing into a plant-based diet. I like this approach because — generally — the longer it takes to get into a habit, the longer it sticks. You can approach a gradual implementation of a plant-based diet in two ways. You want to focus either on what you can eliminate or what you can add in. I'm personally a fan of adding in; it's not as scary as taking something out.

In the next sections, I outline the pros and cons of making a gradual switch. If you decide that a gradual transition is for you, decide whether to eliminate foods or add them. To help you out, I provide some guidelines for both approaches.

Benefits to taking the slow approach

Taking a slow, cautious approach to implementing a plant-based diet means you get the chance to not only absorb the physical and logistical changes that occur but also to slowly digest all the new foods and information along the way. Other advantages include:

✔ You're not as likely to feel anxious that familiar foods have to be taken out of your diet right away. The goal is to focus on adding things in that can help you experience new foods, meals, and recipes and how they impact your body and your overall approach to food.

✔ Your body enjoys the process more as it begins to adjust to fiber, different greens, and seeds. All of these things take time for your body to get used to. Doing this gradually means you won't likely feel harsh detox symptoms, as you would if you went cold turkey.

✔ Your grocery-shopping experiences may be more pleasurable and less stressful than with the cold-turkey approach. You have time to find out about new things, experience them, test them out, and see what sticks and feels right for you. You can also enjoy the process of understanding why plant-based foods are so good for you and your health. It's a whole process, so embrace it with ease.

My own story of going plant-based

I took the gradual approach to become fully plant-based. I eliminated red meat when I was 13, and that set the stage for me to really venture into how I wanted this to become part of my life. After several years, dairy, chicken, and then fish came out of my diet. This gave me a chance to digest and absorb the transitions and changes I was making. I wanted to fully understand what I was doing and how it would serve me. And I did! Now I live and breathe this lifestyle, and it is the approach I use most with my clients, as it's less intimidating and more likely to make sense.

Drawbacks of a slow process

Sometimes when you strive to create new habits, going too slowly can negatively affect your transition. A move to a plant-based diet is no exception, so here's what you should watch out for:

- ✔ You may lack accountability. When you do this process little by little, you may be more likely to fall off the wagon or "cheat." Because you're taking a more relaxed approach, it may be easy to say, "Oh, I'll have my plant-based meal *tomorrow*." Find ways to keep yourself focused on your decision to transition, such as making a calendar that you display on the fridge.

- ✔ You won't feel the expected health benefits right away, and you may give up as a result. You may be hoping to have more energy, get better sleep, and lose weight — but these things take time! You have to motivate yourself until the physical results eventually start to reveal themselves.

- ✔ It's hard to form a new habit for the long term if you haven't given it a solid few weeks of immersion. Experts say it takes 21 days to form a habit. If you go too slowly, you're more likely to deviate from the plan.

- ✔ If you only buy a few new ingredients at a time to restock your pantry, you may find that it's hard to make new recipes. For example, if you don't have the right sweeteners or alternative meat options for your meals, it may be more difficult to make them. A total shift in your pantry can help you make sure you have the ingredients needed to keep you on track.

The process of elimination

When you decide to transition slowly to a plant-based diet, you can take two different paths: You can eliminate non-plant-based foods, or you can add plant-based foods. Of the two gradual approaches, choosing to eliminate non-plant-based foods is probably more difficult. Giving things up that we like and are familiar with is definitely a challenge, but having a plan to phase things out makes it a lot more doable. Everyone is different, and it's important to go with what works for you, but here's the order I recommend for taking foods out of your diet over the course of a few weeks or a few months:

1. **Red meat:** The heaviest of the animal-based foods should only be consumed once in a while. Your body has to work hard to break it down. Look to minimize your intake each week, working toward total elimination. Try consuming red meat only on weekends and reducing further from there.

2. **Chicken and other poultry:** Chicken is a staple in most homes. It's lighter than red meat, so you can start at a higher consumption frequency. Try reducing your poultry intake to three meals a week to start and going down from there.

3. **Fish:** This is the lightest of the animal-flesh foods, but it's not as commonly consumed as poultry. Look at reducing your intake to one to two servings per week and then reducing that intake over time.

4. **Cheese, milk, and other dairy:** This is usually the hardest for people to give up. Most of us have an addiction to dairy. Try to consume dairy foods only one to two times per week until you wean yourself off of them completely. You can find other snacks as alternatives to help you through your transition (more about this in the next section).

Many people still consume dairy on a plant-based diet. If you're among them, I suggest opting for goat- or sheep-derived milks and cheeses. They are cleaner, higher in nutrients, and can be digested by the human body much more easily than cow dairy.

5. **Eggs:** These tend to be a staple for vegetarians, and all I can say to that is, "Everything in moderation." Eggs shouldn't be consumed every day. Save them for special occasions, if at all.

If you want to eliminate foods meal by meal, you can choose one full day each week to go plant-based or choose a few meals throughout the week. Choose days or meals that work well with your lifestyle. For example, you may want to do your plant-based meals on days when you have time to experiment with new recipes, rather than trying to squeeze it in after working late and before the kids' homework time.

The adding-in process

In this process, you focus on adding new items to your diet on a regular basis. Choosing some plant-based essentials helps smooth the transition and give you a healthy and balanced start.

✔ **Green leafy vegetables:** I suggest adding one new green vegetable each week. Also look to add as many leafy greens to as many meals during the day as possible. They nourish you and provide your body with vitamins and minerals. Some examples are spinach, kale, and arugula.

✔ **Non-dairy milk, such as rice or almond milk:** Sometimes, totally switching the milk you drink or put in your cereal is too drastic. You can start transitioning by doing a mix of dairy and non-dairy milk, gradually changing the ratio over time.

✔ **Beans, tofu, tempeh, and quinoa:** Serve these alongside your meat for one or more meals a week or day so you can get used to them, and eventually replace your meat with these options.

✔ **Whole grains:** Experiment by adding different whole grains, such as quinoa, brown rice, and millet, to the base of burgers or meatloaf.

You Can't Do It Alone: Leaning on Others for Support

It's important to know that you don't have to take on these changes to your lifestyle alone. It's always helpful to get support from people around you to make the process that much more rewarding and successful. The following sections outline how you can get the support you need to thrive during this transition.

Surrounding yourself with others who support your lifestyle

You're more likely to be successful if you have people around you who are encouraging you and supporting what you're doing. You may want to have one of the following to turn to, so you can transition to a plant-based diet successfully.

✔ **Community potlucks and meet-ups:** This is a great way to meet people who are on the same journey. They can likely introduce you to new restaurants and markets in the area and to fun activities they participate in as a group. You can find like-minded people online (try www.meetup.com), at vegetarian restaurants, at health-food stores, or through community centers.

✔ **Social-media groups:** Social-media groups provide up-to-date information on plant-based trends and events. Most groups post success stories or highlight role models to follow. This can be a fast avenue to help you get into the plant-based mindset. Good websites to check out include www.happycow.com and www.mindbodygreen.com. If you're into hashtags, do a search for #meatlessmondays, #plantbasedliving, #plantpowered, or #eatplants — just to name a few.

- ✔ **Cooking classes:** Your local community center or health-food store likely has cooking classes at restaurants or other venues. Often, vegetarian websites tell you where local classes are held. (If you live in or are traveling to Toronto, check out my food studio and lifestyle shop, www.marniwasserman.com.)

- ✔ **Friends and family:** Having your family on board or at least interested in your decision can only make the process easier. It's ideal if they're open to trying your new food creations or at least to being supportive of your decision, no matter your reasons.

You may find that some friends and family members aren't receptive or don't understand what you're up to. Resist the urge to become defensive; rather, just trust that you've made a choice that's going to benefit you and your health, and let them worry about the rest. Inspire by example — as you lead, even the naysayers may eventually jump on board to try your new, fun recipes.

Enlisting the help of a nutritionist, naturopath, or medical doctor

When you first make the switch to a plant-based diet, it may be in your best interest to get some support from professionals. They can make sure you're adopting the new lifestyle correctly, answer any questions, and help you see (and celebrate) the changes that take place in your body as a result of eating better. Consider contacting one of these professionals in your area:

- ✔ **Nutritionist:** A nutritionist can help you with food and meal planning. Many can even provide tips on how to overhaul your pantry and fridge and set you up with grocery lists to restock your kitchen. Depending on the nutritionist, you may be able to get customized meal plans and recipes that can help you map out your meals during the week.

  Many nutritionists also work with your overall goals for choosing this lifestyle, whether for weight loss, more energy, better sleep, or what have you. Some can help with natural supplementation to make sure you're getting the nutrients you need to thrive on this diet (see Chapter 9 for more on supplements).

- ✔ **Naturopath:** Working with a natural-medicine doctor can help you address the potential health concerns of changing your diet. Some naturopaths can help with dietary suggestions and meal recommendations, make suggestions regarding allergies and food sensitivities, and even work according to your blood type.

- ✔ **Medical doctor:** You may choose to enlist a medical doctor, and this is especially helpful if you're taking any prescription medications. Your doctor can help you monitor your dosage as you change your diet. You may find that after several months of eating a wholesome, plant-based diet you need less of your medication, and only a doctor can help you with this.

Several medical conditions, such as arthritis, high cholesterol, diabetes, and heart disease, may improve as a result of eating more vegetables. See Chapter 2 for more details.

 Insulin-dependent diabetics who are taking insulin should notify their health-care practitioner before making any dietary changes. Taking the prescribed dose of insulin when that amount is no longer needed can be very dangerous. It's also important that patients never alter or eliminate their medications without consulting their doctor.

Overcoming Common Pitfalls

Part of making a big change in your eating habits is facing challenges and overcoming them. Although everyone is different and has his or her own struggles, it may help to consider these common obstacles and how to tackle them. Half the battle is knowing what to expect and being ready when the time comes. There's nothing you can't surmount!

Having little or no experience in the kitchen

Many people feel like they have to have a culinary education to start eating more healthfully. In my experience with my own clients, people tend to get overwhelmed at the idea of eating more meals at home. Don't let this stop you. When you start anything new — especially when you're taking full responsibility — it can present a challenge. However, you just need to start.

 Get yourself a partner and make a cooking date to start tackling some recipes together. You don't even need a partner who is plant-based — all you need is someone who knows his or her way around a kitchen and may even enjoy giving you some basic help. Make it fun by getting a group together at your house, where everyone can share cooking tips, strategies, and even favorite utensils and tools. Work together and create a meal as a group so you can watch and learn — take notes if you want! Keep it low key and social by making sure the guest list includes your best friends and family.

Another option is to go to a cooking class and get to know other people who are in the same boat. As you build a foundation of basic skills and recipes, you start to feel more confident and willing to take on more challenging recipes. Don't forget to find someone who will be an encouraging taste-tester and cheerleader!

Feeling intimidated by new foods

Quinoa, arame, Swiss chard? These words may feel like a different language to you. That's okay. At one point you didn't know what a tomato, apple, or tangerine was, either. The best thing to do is jump right In.

Start by choosing just a couple of new ingredients that you find in this book (or elsewhere) and do some research on them. Look them up, watch videos on how to prepare them, and find restaurants that serve them so you can experience them before you take them on yourself at home. Don't be afraid to ask questions about how the food is prepared! Practice, experiment, and try all sorts of preparations to find ones you like.

When you feel confident with a food, move on to a new one. New foods (which may actually be ancient varieties) are introduced to the market all the time. Get to know them, and hopefully you'll come to love some of them in new favorite recipes.

Keep your eyes open for "seasonal" or "market" vegetables and fruits on restaurant menus and always order them (especially if you don't know what they are or how to cook them). It's a wonderful, non-threatening way to expand your veggie repertoire while sampling produce at the height of its deliciousness!

Feeling like the odd man out

It can feel strange when you take something on that no one else seems to understand. Sticking to your guns can be especially challenging in social settings, such as going out to restaurants with friends and family members, eating a meal with work colleagues, or even discussing food topics with your neighbors. If you feel strange or awkward, just remember that you've made the decision to take this on for a reason (or many). Instead of feeling left out, you can be inspiring! Be the trendy, cool person who suggests new restaurants or makes a killer tempeh stir-fry. Leading by example can even cause others around you to join in.

As you host dinner parties or go out to eat, it may be helpful to invite a plant-based buddy to join. Maybe it's someone you meet in a cooking class or through an online message board for vegetarians. Or maybe it's a really good friend who goes plant-based for one night to keep you company. Don't be afraid to reach out and ask for help — you're doing a great thing for yourself, and many of your loved ones want to support that. Just tell them how they can.

Be careful not to preach to others that what you're doing is the "right way." This approach only ostracizes folks and makes you seem like . . . well, a know-it-all jerk. And nobody likes that. Instead, be silently content with the way you live and the way you eat. In time, others will come to you with questions.

Fighting food fatigue and boredom

To keep your meals interesting, continue to add new foods, new recipes, and new preparation methods to your repertoire. Even in the non-plant-based world, it's easy to get stuck in a food rut. It's important to expand your horizons — as with anything in life. You can't eat brown rice or veggie burgers every day and feel inspired. Keep trying new cookbooks, new cooking classes, and new restaurants. Go to different stores to do your shopping.

You don't always have to change up the food itself; you can find many ways to prepare the same food, so experiment with different techniques and seasonings. For example, try steamed kale with garlic and olive oil one night as a side dish, but the next day try baked kale chips with sea salt as a snack! And don't be afraid to "go off book" — that is, you can use recipes as loose guides but add your own spin to keep your meals lively and interesting.

It's always nice to go to farmers' markets and specialty shops, as they usually have a high changeover of product and also work with the season. You're virtually guaranteed to see things you haven't seen before. This may push you outside your comfort zone to get reconnected to your plant-based goals and excited about new food items.

Chapter 6

Looking at What's on Your Plate

Discussions about good nutrition, lessons about healthy habits, and thoughts about wellness are important to building a foundation for your plant-based lifestyle, but here's where the fork meets the mouth. At the end of the day, it comes down to the choices you make and what goes on your plate. So make sure you build your plate with nourishing plant-based foods.

In this chapter, I give you some specific points to keep in mind about the foods you choose, offer some alternatives to the three-squares-a-day meal approach, and outline some sample menus to get you started on your new plant-based lifestyle. I also suggest ways to convert some of your favorite foods into plant-based favorites.

Thinking about Your New Plate

When you look at your plate from now on, I hope it's as bright and bountiful as mine! Your plate at every meal should be loaded with a balance of wholesome plant-based foods that are both nutritious and delicious. Read on to learn how you can create a plate that satisfies your taste buds and supports your health.

Keeping it whole

Choosing foods that are as wholesome and real as possible is the first step to achieving nourishing meals. What do I mean by "real" foods? I mean foods that are in their natural forms and not packaged or processed. Not only are processed foods filled with additives, excess salts, sugars, and preservatives (even if they're vegetarian), but it's also harder for you to control how much of them you're eating.

Choosing organic over nonorganic

When it comes to choosing produce, you want to choose organic wherever and whenever possible. This ensures that you're putting the highest quality foods into your body. Organic produce hasn't been sprayed with pesticides, fungicides, or herbicides, which are used to kill pests and diseases. If those substances kill them, what are they doing to you?

Buying organic also means that the produce has been grown in soil that is well maintained with nutrients, which results in fruits and vegetables that ultimately have more nutrients and taste better. I would suggest making an effort to choose as much organic produce as possible. To find out which ones to start with, check out the lists in Chapter 8.

However, if you make your own snacks and meals, you can manage your portion sizes more effectively, and you know the foods come from clean, healthy sources. For example, instead of eating a canned veggie medley as a side for your dinner, opt for buying your own whole organic carrots from the produce section at the grocery store and roasting them yourself.

Dishing it up in the right proportions

Ideally, you should keep your plate proportionate. Try to maintain certain ratios of different plant-based foods so you get enough protein, carbohydrates, and fats to nourish you at every meal. Ideally, you want to feel like your meal will sustain you, which means having eaten enough food to feel energized and being able to wait two to three hours before eating your next meal. At the end of the day (literally), you want to feel satisfied — because you ate from each food category and are nourished from the inside out. Just note that my definition of "feeling nourished" may not align with yours, so really pay attention to what feels best for you and adjust accordingly.

Figure 6-1 shows what your typical plate should look like. A majority of the plate is made up of vegetables because they are the mainstays of a plant-based diet. However, you want to choose the right balance of vegetables so you'll be sustained and full after each meal. Root vegetables and green leafies should make up most of your plate. From there grains, beans, and legumes will fill up the rest of your plate. If you can begin to mentally divide your plate at each meal to look like the one in Figure 6-1 (more or less), then you are taking a large step toward success at a plant-based lifestyle.

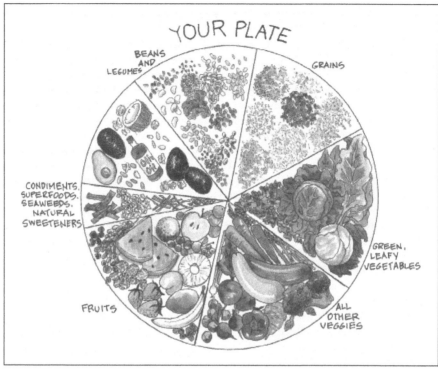

YOUR PLATE

BEANS AND LEGUMES

GRAINS

CONDIMENTS, SUPERFOODS, SEAWEEDS, NATURAL SWEETENERS

GREEN, LEAFY VEGETABLES

FRUITS

ALL OTHER VEGGIES

Figure 6-1:
It's all about
the right
proportions!

Illustration by Elizabeth Kurtzman

A word about fruit

Figure 6-1 shows fruit on the plate. However, that may not represent how your lunch or dinner plate will look. Instead, it gives you an idea of how your meals should be balanced over the course of a day.

You generally want to eat a majority of your fruit in the morning, for a snack, or on its own in between meals. Doing so allows for optimal digestion and energy. However, fruit may be combined with other foods, such as in a smoothie (with a brown rice protein or pea powder, green leafy vegetables, coconut oil, a sprinkling of sea vegetables, and some superfoods) or a breakfast cereal or porridge.

Don't think that you must have a serving of fruit on your plate at every meal, because that can wreak havoc on your digestion. Fruit contains simple sugars that digest quite rapidly, so when fruit is combined with too many foods, it can leave you gassy and bloated. The best way to consume fresh fruit is to eat whole single fruits with minimal other foods or blend it in a smoothie, which makes the fruit easier to digest.

When you take fruit off the plate when planning a larger meal, you can fill that void with green leafy or root vegetables, whole grains, or beans.

Consuming calories that count

Calories. Most of us are all too familiar with these little guys as something to count and avoid. But they do serve an actual purpose beyond torment-ing us — they measure the approximate amount of energy needed to raise the temperature of one gram of water by one degree. We use this measure to understand how food "adds up" or is stored in our body and how it's metabolized.

In my eyes, when it comes to counting calories, it's most definitely not about the *amount* of calories but more about *the source* of those calories. When you focus strictly on the caloric values of foods, you stop paying attention to what is actually in them (the good and bad nutrients). Now, I'm not tell-ing you to completely overlook the caloric content, but I *am* saying that the number of calories isn't as relevant as the actual nutrients. So let's talk about how to get good calories that are nutritious!

Getting your calories from whole foods is the first step. Whether you're eating grains, seeds and nuts, beans, or fruits and veggies, strive to eat fresh foods from whole sources that don't come out of a package. (Of course, pack-aged products may find their way into your life from time to time, which is okay. There are many health foods that come in a package.) It's your job to look closely at what you're eating, whether it comes in a package or not, and ultimately be conscious about the calories you take in.

It comes down to how your food impacts you nutritionally, not calorically. For example, a single serving of junk food, such as chips, bagels, or cookies, easily contains way more than 200 calories. The nutritional value of these foods is next to zero. However, if you consume 200 calories in a single serv-ing of plant-based foods such as nuts, seeds, quinoa, avocados, or coconut, for example, you're much better off. These foods provide your body with nourishment from protein, healthy fat, and complex carbohydrates. So you're likely to feel satisfied more quickly, and you may even consume fewer calo-ries because your body is using the nutrients. With junk food, you can pretty much eat endlessly with nothing to show for it except maybe a pair of jeans that doesn't fit anymore.

Table 6-1 shows how 200 calories of common foods stack up against one another. Notice how much of the plant-based foods you can eat (approxi-mately) compared to a junk-food equivalent.

Table 6-1	Comparison of 200 Calories in Plant-Based Food versus Junk Food	
Plant-Based Food	*Junk Food*	
2 to 3 apples	1 small (2.5 ounces or 72 grams) blueberry muffin	
One 4.4-ounce (125-gram) avocado	1 handful (1.4 ounces or 41 grams) of chips	
2 heads (21 ounces or 588 grams) of broccoli	Half (1.4 ounces or 41 grams) of a chocolate bar	
2 bunches (50 ounces or 1,425 grams) of celery stalks	Half of a side serving (2.6 ounces or 73 grams) of french fries	

You need to look at your food calories more critically and decide how you want to gain the most nutrition from your food.

Eliminating refined processed foods from your diet

It may be daunting to kick a habit that you've gotten so used to — especially if you don't even realize that you have it — but kicking refined processed foods (such as junk food) out of your diet is a worthy cause to take up. They make up a significant amount of your caloric intake without giving you the nutrition you deserve, so they definitely need to go.

Once upon a time, our grandparents and great-grandparents didn't have the option to eat processed food. All they had was fresh, minimally processed foods. Nowadays, fresh food can be hard to come by, especially because of the convenience of processed foods and the lack of knowledge about how they negatively impact your health.

To keep food in packages, manufacturers often need to add "foodlike substances" to make them last longer or taste better. These enhancers make processed foods even worse for you, so what you're left with is a processed food containing food stabilizers, preservatives, added sugar, and salt. Who wants that? Consciously, of course, it sounds horrible, but the trouble is that you may already be addicted (like so many of us are). As a plant-based eater, you want to source only the best possible foods that enhance your health — and that means staying away from refined processed foods.

Try these pointers to start kicking your refined-food habit:

- **Shop with a plan, not with an empty stomach.** When you're hungry, you lose your judgment and basically want to put anything you see in your mouth! So plan ahead — not only in terms of having a shopping list but also making sure you have some food in your belly.

- **Stock up on fiber.** Fiber-rich whole foods fill you up and are the nutritional opposite of refined foods, which have been stripped of their fiber.

- **Swap out sugared drinks for homemade brews.** This is a sure-fire way to drop calories within moments. Just a few sips of a processed fruit juice or soda can add a significant amount of non-nutritive calories before you've even eaten a meal. Make ginger or peppermint tea, or throw some fresh berries in a bottle of water.

- **Avoid fast foods like the plague.** Fast food is quite possibly the worst thing you can eat, because most menus are loaded with fat and calories. Set yourself up for success by always having enough food on hand to make quick meals. Plan ahead by making a little extra for dinner so you can have leftovers the next day.

- **Try some good things that come in packages.** Some whole foods, such as grains, nuts, and seeds, require packaging to keep them on a shelf. This is okay; just be sure you check the dates on the packages.

    These common plant-based snacks are wrapped up and ready to go:

    - Brown-rice cakes
    - Coconut yogurt
    - Dairy-free dark-chocolate bars
    - Unsulphured dried fruit and nut bars
    - Granola and other whole-grain cereals
    - Kale chips
    - Organic corn chips
    - Plant-based protein powder
    - Trail mixes
    - Whole-grain or gluten-free crackers

Maintaining proper hydration

Hydration is an important but often neglected subject. The body is made up of about 60 percent water, and yet many people don't drink nearly as much as they should to keep their bodies well hydrated. Many plants are made up mostly of water, which is good news for plant-based eaters, but you still need to down some good-quality (preferably filtered) H_2O several times a day.

If you aren't hydrated, your body can't metabolize, process, and function at its best. By the time you feel thirsty, you're already dehydrated. When you're dehydrated, you can experience everything from fatigue to headaches to cramping.

Drink water throughout the day. Whether it's plain water, lemon water, or herbal tea, just make sure to get it in. Opinions differ on how much you should drink, but a typical recommendation is to drink half your body weight in ounces; if you weigh 150 pounds, you should drink about 75 ounces (about nine cups) of water a day. This may not be realistic, but at least make sure you're drinking something — and that doesn't mean coffee or other caffeinated beverages (because these can dehydrate your body further).

Be careful about drinking too much water at meals. Diluting your stomach acids can impair digestion.

People often wonder whether they should drink bottled water or tap water. This is an ongoing source of research and controversy. On one hand, you have water that is being stored in a plastic bottle, which can leach all kinds of toxins into the water, and who really knows the source? On the other hand, do you trust your local water treatment plant to filter the water that comes through your pipes to the point that it's pure enough for your drinking pleasure? Most city water and even rural water isn't as clean as we'd like to think; debris, waste, and agricultural runoff all leak into our water systems.

The best solution is to buy your own filters so that most of what you're consuming is clean. Search online to find the filtration system that's best for you. You can place a simple one on your faucet, invest in a triple filter installed beneath the sink, or use anything in between.

Going with Your Gut

Your gut isn't just for digestion and metabolizing your foods. It's also that little voice inside you that tells you when something is right or wrong. You can use that as your navigation system when trying to reach your nutrition goals, eat the right amounts, or choose the right foods for the right reasons.

Eating intuitively

Intuitive eating is an approach that involves listening to your body to determine whether you're actually hungry, craving something, or just plain bored. This may sound like a far-reaching concept for some, because many people eat strictly from a survival standpoint or select foods based solely on taste as opposed to choosing things at the right time. People often eat according to the "three square meals a day" approach without realizing whether they're really hunger or eating just because it's the right time of day. Getting in touch with what's really going on with your hunger helps you make the right food choices at the right times.

Consider these tips for intuitive eating:

- ✔ **When you crave junk food, stop before you act.** Identify what you really want and figure out whether you can reach for something plant-based instead.

- ✔ **When you're eating your delicious, hearty plant-based meal and are starting to feel full, stop.** Give your brain time to catch up with your stomach to determine whether you really need those last few bites. A lot of us are trained to stuff ourselves past the point of full or to clean our plates, but that's not always the best idea. Listen to yourself, and you may find that you want to set the rest aside for later when you're actually hungry.

- ✔ **Eat only when you're truly hungry, as opposed to eating just because you're on a schedule or timeline.** You may find that your body naturally allows you to eat when it wants to, not when you think it should.

Managing your metabolism

A lot of people want to manage their metabolism, but most don't know how and inadvertently do all the wrong things — or worse, they *think* they understand it, but they don't. (For my purposes here, *metabolism* refers to the chemical reactions that occur in the body, including digestion and the transport of substances into and between different cells.) Things like not eating regular meals or eating the wrong balance of food can slow down your metabolism, cause weight gain, and make you feel tired and generally unwell.

Here are some of the best ways to manage your metabolism:

- ✔ **Eat four to six regular meals throughout the day.** Three of these meals can be slightly larger meals, and the others can be smaller snacks.

- ✔ **Maintain your plant protein intake with complex carbohydrates.** Keep up with your beans, nuts, and seeds along with whole grains, sweet potatoes, vegetables, and fruits. These foods can help keep you satisfied between meals and keep your metabolism burning.

✔ **Drink lots of water.** Dehydration can slow down your resting metabolic rate. Without water going through your body, you can't flush things out. There isn't an exact amount you should drink, but keep hydrated all day long, even if that means carrying a water bottle. You know you're properly hydrated when your urine is pale yellow or almost clear.

✔ **Add a shot of apple-cider vinegar to your routine.** A tablespoon of apple-cider vinegar added to a glass of water can boost your metabolism. If you take it first thing in the morning, it can also help your body eliminate waste and help with digestion. Apple-cider vinegar is used in many fat-flush and weight-loss diets, but some people take it to an extreme. Give this tip a try once in a while, because it really can work wonders when it comes to your metabolism.

✔ **Drink warm lemon water in the morning and sip green tea during the day.** Starting your day with ½ cup of warm water mixed with 2 tablespoons of fresh-squeezed lemon juice helps regulate and jump-start your digestive tract. It gets your digestive juices going, helps your body eliminate waste, and makes you feel more energized. Green tea can help increase metabolic rate while also improving fat oxidation. So enjoy one to two cups a day.

✔ **Exercise.** Nothing helps boost your metabolism like exercise. The more you move your body, the more calories you burn. Also, the more strength-training exercise you do and the more muscle mass you build, the more your body keeps metabolizing calories all day long.

Many people have a glass of ice water with their meals. This can be problematic for digestion. Consuming too much water with food can dilute stomach acids and enzymes and prevent digestion from happening. Instead, drink a glass or two of room temperature water about 30 minutes before you eat and then again one to two hours after your meal. However, you can still sip water as you eat to help get the food down.

Getting Organized

The first step to meal planning and the one that most people have the most difficulty with is organizing meals for the week. If you don't plan ahead, you can set yourself up for falling off track, eating the wrong foods, or, even worse, missing a meal. To help prevent this, use meal planning to set yourself up for successful eating all week long. The following sections explain how to plan a week's worth of meals and how to use that meal plan to create a list of ingredients you need from the grocery store.

Understanding the importance of meal planning

Meal planning, whether it's just for you or for your whole family, can be challenging and overwhelming. Even if you intend to eat only healthy foods, it's easy for your lifestyle and other excuses to get in the way. Maybe you work late, or you forget to pack a lunch. Maybe you just don't have time to grocery shop. At the end of the day, you're hungry and prone to ordering in or going out for dinner, where the choices aren't always as nutritious as what you can cook for yourself.

The best way to get started with meal planning is to make a chart with the days of the week written across the top and the meals listed down the side. You can base the columns on either five days or seven days (sometimes people like to leave the weekends up for grabs without planning). Then create four to six rows to account for breakfast, lunch, and dinner and two to three snacks in between.

After you've created your chart, select the recipes or foods you want to serve each day and plug them into the plan. Check out the recipes in Chapters 10–15 for some great ideas.

You may want to focus on some of the guidelines mentioned in the earlier "Dishing it up in the right proportions" section to create balanced meals. In that case, you need to figure out how many items you need to make per meal or what foods you need to add to make sure to get your green veggies, grains, and beans. You may want to make a well-rounded recipe, or you can simply add a side to complement the main dish. For instance, say the main part of your meal is going to be the Warm Festive Farro Salad from Chapter 12. You may want to pair it with a side of steamed greens, a side of white beans, or some hummus. When you mix and match different dishes, you'll become more creative and discover which combinations of plant-based items make up a balanced meal.

You don't have to make a new dish every day for every meal. Prepare extra food and use the leftovers to maximize your meals and your time.

For new ideas and recipes, subscribe to a recipe-focused blog, website (like Pinterest), newsletter, or magazine. Or get a slew of plant-based cookbooks that you can rotate through.

Later in this chapter, I provide you with some simple, delicious meal ideas that can help you prepare for your busy week. But first, try these tips to help you follow a meal plan:

✔ Do your grocery shopping on the weekend for easy meal preparation throughout the week.

✔ Make at least two main dishes on the weekend or at the beginning of the week, along with one or two batches of soup and small salads or dips for the week (see Part III for all kinds of recipe ideas).

✔ Make one or two new recipes midweek (if time permits) for variety.

✔ Have on hand a variety of on-the-go snacks, such as trail mix, nut and seed bars, cut-up veggies, and bean dip.

✔ Get yourself equipped with a cooler/cold pack and to-go containers.

Making your plant-based grocery list

So how do you make a good grocery list? Well, the first thing you need is pen and paper. No, seriously. To have an effective list, you need to either write it down or create it on your phone or computer (there are even special apps for that) — whichever way works best for you. In Chapter 7, I give you a complete list of plant-based items to stock up on, so refer to that for more specifics on *what* to get. Here I'm talking about *how* to make your list.

First, it helps to determine into which shopper category you naturally fall:

✔ **The organizer:** This person likes to be on top of things and knows what to expect. You methodically go through each of the food categories (grains, proteins, vegetables, fruits, oils and fats, and superfoods) every week and write down what you need. Even if you don't think you need anything, you go through the process anyway to make sure nothing is missed. This is a good approach for beginner plant-based foodies, because you can visualize which foods are in which category, and it also helps you navigate the grocery store in an efficient manner.

✔ **The shopper by recipe:** This means you select a few recipes you want to make for the week and make a list based on them specifically. So, in essence, you just buy what your recipes call for.

✔ **The on-the-fly shopper:** This describes someone who wants to take a chance, walk around, and grab things as she sees them. Likely this is someone creative who can work with whatever food items she has on hand.

✔ **The list runner:** This person keeps a running list of items he runs out of, perhaps on his counter or fridge. He looks at and adds to it constantly. If you fall into this category, you typically have a mental idea of what you need to get and what you have already, and you may just need to make an additional mini list of "extras." Likely, you're well stocked to begin with because of regular grocery-store trips and just need things like produce or specialty items.

After you determine what type of shopper you are, formulate your grocery list. Write down what you need and then hit the grocery store.

Not making a list can set you up for not-so-good results. When you don't make a list, you may buy random, unwanted items that waste your time and money, among other things. Consider these three consequences of not making a good list:

- **You overbuy on items you already have.** It's important to take an inventory of items at home; otherwise, you may end up with foods well past their expiration date.

- **You buy unhealthy or unwanted ingredients,** kind of like impulse buying the latest gadget or trendy article of clothing. You may think you want it, but it's not really in your plans for the week — again, just wasted money.

- **You don't get what you want or anything at all.** Without a proper plan, you may get overwhelmed at the store and be too intimidated to buy anything at all, resulting in a wasted trip and an empty shopping bag.

Exploring Sample Meal Plans

Now that you have the tools to make a great list (see the preceding section), make sure you get yourself on track each day with a good, solid meal plan. These sample meal plans for breakfast, lunch, dinner, and snacks can help you get started. After that, I go into more-specific plans to help you meet your goals as a new plant-based eater.

Breakfast ideas

Add these ideas to your list to start your day off right (see Chapter 10 for even more):

- **One or two slices of sprouted-grain toast with your nut butter of choice and sliced banana,** along with a glass of rice milk (with or without a scoop of protein powder).

- **Half a cup of cooked whole-grain porridge (oats, quinoa, spelt, or buckwheat) cooked with almond or rice milk.** Add in dried fruits, such as cranberries, apricots, or raisins; fresh fruits, such as blueberries; nuts, such as almonds, walnuts, or pecans; or seeds, such as pumpkin, sunflower, flax, hemp, or chia.

✔ **Fresh fruit or green smoothie** made of one to two cups of rice, almond, hemp, or coconut milk. Add in banana, berries, ground chia or flaxseeds, a scoop of plant-based protein powder, and a handful of spinach or kale.

Lunch and dinner options

Keep your menu (and belly) full with these meal ideas (more recipes in Chapters 11 and 12):

✔ **Power-packed salad** with a base of romaine, leaf lettuce, or arugula. Add in:

- **Veggie protein:** ¼ to ½ cup chickpeas, kidney beans, black beans, lima beans, or marinated tempeh or tofu

- **Raw or steamed veggies:** Carrots, bell peppers, celery, beets, cucumbers, tomatoes, onions, spinach, or sprouts

- **Healthy fat:** Avocados, olives, olive oil, hempseed oil, nuts, and seeds

- **Soaked or toasted sea vegetables:** Arame, wakame, dulse, or nori (for a refresher on these, see Chapter 4)

- **Fresh or dried fruit:** Apple, pear, strawberries, raspberries, dried cranberries, raisins, or currants

- **Extras:** ½ cup cooked whole grain or beans, quinoa, brown rice, barley, millet, or lentils (for more on grains, head back to Chapter 3)

✔ **Sandwich with whole-grain, sprouted-grain, or gluten-free bread or a wrap** loaded with hummus, avocados, sprouts, veggies, and lettuce.

✔ **Soup with chunky veggies or a pureed vegetable soup.**

- **Base:** Water and dried herbs, miso paste, or homemade vegetable broth

- **Veggies:** Celery, carrots, onions, broccoli, kale, spinach, bok choy, cauliflower, asparagus, or zucchini

- **Beans:** Chickpeas, black beans, white beans, lentils, or split peas

- **Starchy veggies:** Sweet potatoes or squash

- **Whole grains:** Barley, brown rice, or quinoa

- **Sea veggies:** Dulse, arame, wakame, or nori

Macronutrients plate

You can create an entire meal from nothing but wholesome sides. A good selection of sides can become a full meal that is hearty and nourishing. (You basically create the plate shown in Figure 6-1, but without the fruit category.) Mix and match foods from the following categories:

- **Cooked whole grains:** Millet, buckwheat, brown rice, spelt, kamut, quinoa, or brown-rice pasta
- **Starchy vegetables (steamed, roasted, or grilled):** Squash, carrots, beans, parsnips, sweet potatoes, or acorn squash
- **Steamed or sautéed veggies:** Broccoli, kale, green beans, bok choy, Swiss chard, collards, mushrooms, onions, bell peppers, eggplant, zucchini, snap peas, or asparagus
- **Organic tofu, tempeh, or beans** (marinated, baked, grilled, stewed, or steamed)
- **Fats:** Avocados, olive oil, coconut oil, nuts, or seeds
- **Condiments:** Tamari, olive oil, lemon juice, apple-cider vinegar, seaweed, and herbs and spices

Snacks

In between meals, you'll want to keep yourself fueled with snacks or mini-meals. Try one or two of these suggestions:

- Whole-grain crackers or brown-rice cakes with nut or seed butter
- Fresh fruit
- Trail mix (try the Super Brazil and Goldenberry Trail Mix recipe in Chapter 14)
- A homemade muffin (see the Apple Cinnamon Mini-Muffins recipe in Chapter 10)
- Hummus or bean dip with brown-rice crackers or sliced veggies (check out the Edamame Hummus recipe in Chapter 14)
- Guacamole with corn chips (see the Sweet Pea Guacamole recipe in Chapter 14)
- Homemade energy bar
- A smoothie (try the Chocolate Banana Super Smoothie recipe in Chapter 14 or the Liquid Nutrition Smoothie in Chapter 10)

Light meals for weight loss

I don't promote dieting per se, because I strongly believe that if you eat the right things in balance, you naturally achieve a healthy weight. That being said, choosing certain foods over others helps you get to your goals a little bit more quickly. Table 6-2 shows some lighter options for meals.

Table 6-2	Weight-Loss Meal Plan		
Breakfast (see Chapter 10 for recipes)	**Lunch (see Chapter 11 for recipes)**	**Snack (see Chapter 14 for recipes)**	**Dinner (see Chapter 12 for recipes)**
1–2 cups Liquid Nutrition Smoothie	Kale and Cabbage Slaw with ¼ avocado and topped with a handful of sprouts	Apple or pear with a handful of walnuts or 1 tablespoon of almond butter	Hearty Vegetable Cacciatore with or without ½ cup brown-rice pasta and a large green salad
1 cup Soaked Oats with Goji Berries	1–2 cups of Citrus Wild Rice and Broccoli served over spinach	Brown-rice cake with almond butter	Tangy Tempeh Teriyaki Stir-Fry with ½ cup brown rice
½–1 cup Morning Millet Granola with Homemade Hempseed Milk	Nori roll with a green salad	Carrot and celery sticks with ½ cup Edamame Hummus or Sweet Pea Guacamole	1–2 slices of Mushroom and Chickpea Loaf on a bed of steamed greens topped with 1 tablespoon of Tahini-Miso Gravy (see Chapter 15)

Punches of protein

Whether you train hard at the gym or just find that you feel better eating more protein, you may want to follow a meal plan that looks like the one in Table 6-3. However, be sure to rotate these items regularly with other high-protein plant-based foods.

Table 6-3	Protein-Filled Meal Plan		
Breakfast (see Chapter 10 for recipes)	*Lunch (see Chapter 11 for recipes)*	*Snack (see Chapter 14 for recipes)*	*Dinner (see Chapter 12 for recipes)*
1 cup Turmeric Tofu Scramble with a slice of sprouted-grain toast and ¼ avocado	1–2 cups Quinoa Tabbouleh Salad	½ cup Super Brazil and Goldenberry Trail Mix	Tangy Tempeh Teriyaki Stir-Fry on a bed of brown-rice noodles or wild rice
1–2 cups Liquid Nutrition Smoothie with a full scoop of protein	Hearty sand-wich with tempeh, avocado, and sprouts, plus a large salad	1 Happy Hemp Loaf	Black Bean Cumin Burger with a Kale and Cabbage Slaw Salad, sliced avocado, and Garlic Oregano Yam Fries
½ cup Soaked Oats with Goji Berries with additional plant-based protein mixed in	New Age Minestrone with a green salad or 1 slice of sprouted-grain toast	1–2 cups Chocolate Banana Super Smoothie	Maple-marinated tofu, red citrus spinach quinoa, and steamed broccoli
Super Chia Banana Porridge	Large bowl of Kale and Cabbage Slaw Salad topped with avocado, sprouts, and chickpeas	1–2 Apple Cinnamon Bites with 1 cup almond milk or Homemade Hempseed Milk (see Chapter 10)	Warm Festive Farro Salad with sautéed collard greens with garlic and olive oil

Foods for energy and endurance

You don't have to be athletic to want energy all day long. The meal ideas in Table 6-4 are balanced and well rounded to keep you sustained with nutrients to keep you going.

Table 6-4	Energy-Boosting Meal Plan		
Breakfast (see Chapter 10 for recipes)	*Lunch (see Chapter 11 for recipes)*	*Snack (see Chapter 14 for recipes)*	*Dinner (see Chapter 12 for recipes)*
Super Chia Banana Porridge	Ultimate sandwich with Edamame Hummus	1–2 cups Chocolate Banana Super Smoothie	Arame Soba Noodle Salad with a cup of Chunky Miso Soup
2 Blueberry Buckwheat Pancakes with fresh fruit and 1–2 tablespoons of nut butter	1–2 cups Quinoa Tabbouleh Salad	1–2 Apple Cinnamon Bites	Sweet Potato Shepherd's Pie with steamed kale
1 cup Soaked Oats with Goji Berries	Bowl of Chunky Miso Soup or New Age Minestrone with a side salad with olive oil and vinegar	1 apple with Almond Butter and Cinnamon Dip (see Chapter 15)	Warm Festive Farro Salad on a bed of spinach topped with ¼ cup white beans
Liquid Nutrition Smoothie	Sun Seed Nori Rolls with 1 cup or more of Kale and Cabbage Slaw Salad	1 rice cake topped with tahini, Edamame Hummus, or Sweet Pea Guacamole	1–2 cups Zesty Pesto Pasta with White Beans and a green salad

Modifying Your Favorite Recipes to Be Plant-Based

You may be thinking, "It's all well and good to learn about these new foods and how to prepare them, but what about my old favorite comfort foods?" You know the ones I mean — the ones you're afraid you'll miss so much that you'll just *have* to cheat on your plant-based diet. They're the ones that are so good, you feel certain there isn't a plant-based alternative. Well, I can't think of even one food that I haven't been able to modify in the plant-based world. Everything from chili to chocolate cake can be made with wholesome and natural ingredients.

Try these tips for modifying common comfort foods. In Chapter 7, I get even deeper into detail on how to swap common non-plant-based ingredients for plant-based ones.

- ✔ **Chili:** Because chili is a vegetable-dense meal, you just have to swap out the ground meat. Adding extra protein from kidney beans or black beans is a great choice.

- ✔ **Chocolate cake:** Replace the milk, eggs, and butter with non-dairy milks, ground chia seeds, and coconut oil.

- ✔ **Pizza:** Make crusts from whole-grain flour and use toppings such as nuts, seeds, avocados, and nutritional yeast — among other creative ideas.

- ✔ **Macaroni and cheese:** Revamp this comforting childhood classic with gluten-free brown-rice noodles and a sauce made from butternut squash and tahini.

- ✔ **Meat and potatoes:** Make a hearty dish with portobello mushrooms, tempeh, or tofu instead, with a side of Rosemary Cauliflower Mashed Potatoes (see Chapter 15 for the recipe), sweet potatoes, or squash.

Serve some of these new plant-based dishes alongside your old favorites. This may help you ease the transition to a plant-based lifestyle and show you just how delicious and satisfying plant-based foods can be! (See Chapter 5 for more about transitioning to a plant-based diet.)

Chapter 7

Overhauling Your Kitchen Contents

. . . .

In This Chapter

▶ Making room in your kitchen for your new plant-based diet

▶ Figuring out plant-based foods and grocery lists to get you started

▶ Taking inventory of the essential utensils and equipment

. . . .

*I*t's time to renovate your kitchen, plant-based style! This chapter guides you through the basics of getting rid of what doesn't belong anymore and restocking with plant-based goodness. Although this undertaking may be a little scary because you have to start letting go of some long-time habits and food friends, it's also a really fun adventure because you get to make a fresh start and buy new things (and who doesn't like buying new things?).

This is all about feeling confident in your kitchen — when you have all the supplies (including food and utensils) you need, you're much more likely to be inspired to spend time in your kitchen to make delicious plant-based meals. This chapter tells you what foods and utensils to keep on hand.

Cleaning Out Your Kitchen

As with any new undertaking, it's out with the old before it's in with the new, so the first step is to clean up your kitchen and make some room for all the new goodies you need to stock! Look at your fridge, your pantry, and any other places where you store unhealthy, packaged, and processed food — and remove anything that doesn't fit into a plant-based lifestyle. Just follow these easy steps:

✔ **Get rid of the junk.** There's a good chance your pantry is like mine once was — loaded with a wide variety of chips, crackers, cookies, and cereals that need to be expelled because they're loaded with sugar, salt, and fat — so start there. Then move on to your fridge, where you probably have jams, peanut butter, condiments, salad dressings, and fruit juices, all of which can be discarded. As hard as it is, letting go of your ties to these foods is super important — not just so you can more easily adjust to a plant-based diet but also so you can live better! Although you may think your old faithful foods make your life happier or healthier, I can assure you that most things in your cupboard are only sabotaging you.

The bottom line is that you want to get rid of any foods that don't naturally come from the ground, meaning they're as wholesome as possible. This includes all meats (look in your freezer), eggs, and dairy products, as well as refined flours and pastas, canned goods, and processed cooking oils, such as canola oil and generic vegetable oil.

Low-fat popcorn, granola bars, and 100-calorie pudding cups don't count as healthy plant-based snacks — toss 'em!

✔ **Dump or donate.** Anything that is open needs to go directly into the garbage. Unopened, unexpired food can go to a food bank — use your discretion on what to donate. Otherwise, just dump it! If it's not good for you, chances are it's not better for anyone else to consume. Junk food is junk food! That doesn't mean you can't treat yourself every now and then, but don't keep it in your kitchen, as that is just setting you up for temptation and an unhealthy choice down the road. Take initiative and dump it.

✔ **Get over it.** After detoxing your cupboards, you may be a bit sad and worried that you have nothing left to eat. I can assure you that is absolutely not true. You can find a healthy, wholesome, and tasty alternative to everything you got rid of. Trust me, I don't believe in tasteless food or dieting. I believe in whole, fresh, and delicious food, which is what you need from now on. You'll be satisfied and content when you have a kitchen that is loaded with incredibly delicious food. Just keep reminding yourself that it's all going to be okay — I promise!

✔ **Restock.** Now is the time to get to the market and stock back up. You can find pretty much everything you need at your local health-food or grocery store. Most stores now have sections that are just bursting with natural, fresh, and organic products. Get ahold of cereals that are high in fiber and low in sugar, cookies that are sweetened with fruit juice, and crackers with sea salt (not table salt). Experiment with whole grains, flours, breads, and pastas like spelt, oat, kamut, or quinoa (more on those grains in Chapter 3) instead of wheat-based products. Buy almond butter instead of peanut butter, apple butter instead of jam, maple syrup instead of sugar, coconut oil instead of canola oil, and rolled oats instead of quick oats. Lastly, make sure your fridge is brimming full of fresh fruits and vegetables; that way you always have something to snack on and add to any meal.

I know it can be overwhelming, but just take small steps, and soon you'll have a kitchen stocked with the best foods, and you'll feel inspired to prepare more foods at home. And don't forget that with your kitchen freshly made over, you just happen to be making over your health, too.

Creating Your Plant-Based Starter Kit

The plant-based world — as you probably know by now — is extremely diverse and filled with a lot of variety. There are certain foods that you want to get a head start with right away. These items are not only saturated with flavor but also chock-full of protein (and that certain something that many folks miss when they cut out meat). All the options I describe in the following sections give your body the nutrition it needs (and possibly craves) — plus, they taste good!

Tempeh

Tempeh is a traditional Indonesian food made by splitting, cooking, and fermenting soybeans. It looks like a textured piece of tofu but is more versatile than tofu. Tempeh's hearty texture holds bold flavors and lends itself to veggie burgers, kabobs, salads, and stir-fries.

- **Benefits:** Tempeh is an energy-building food. Tempeh also contains protein and omega-3 fatty acids. The most unique feature is that it's held together by enzymes that make it easy to digest because of its probiotics. Tempeh also gives your body much-needed B vitamins. If you make your own (check out *Fermenting For Dummies* to find out how), it's an amazing source of B12.

- **Where to find it:** You'll likely find tempeh in the freezer or refrigerated section of most grocery stores. It often comes in different flavors with different herbs, seeds, or grains added. I prefer to eat it plain.

- **Where to store it:** I recommend buying only one to three packs at a time to keep it fresh. It's best stored in your freezer.

Talking about tofu

You've likely heard of tofu, a popular form of soy. Tofu is actually soybeans pressed into a block. I like to call it the "cheese" of soy, because it looks like a block of cheese. It comes in a package and can be purchased at most grocery stores. Just be sure you purchase an organic and non-GMO version of tofu (it's even better if it's sprouted). This ensures the best quality and minimal processing.

Tofu is an incredible source of protein and calcium. It can be used in place of meat in many recipes because it will take on any flavor you want. You can cut it into cubes, slices, or triangles, or even grind it up for some texture. Eat it in moderation (no more than a few times a week), just like anything else in your diet.

Quinoa

Quinoa is a high-energy *pseudo-grain* (one of the seeds and grasses we commonly categorize as grain) and a complete protein. It's small and comes in whitish-yellow, red, and black varieties. It's a complete protein with an essential amino-acid profile similar to milk, and it contains more calcium than milk. It's high in lysine, which is scarce in the vegetable kingdom, and rich in vital vitamins and minerals, such as iron, phosphorus, B vitamins, and vitamin E.

Quinoa is so easy to prepare that it typically quickly becomes a favorite, regardless of one's culinary preferences. Quinoa is as versatile as rice and can be substituted into many recipes that call for rice, millet, or couscous.

- ✔ **Benefits:** Quinoa is a pseudo-grain that is easy to digest, making it an excellent endurance and fitness food. It is strengthening to the whole body, but especially to the kidneys and heart. Quinoa has the highest protein content of any pseudo-grain (16 percent), and it has an excellent amino-acid profile.

- ✔ **Where to find it:** You'll find it at most stores in the grain or dry-goods sections. It can be found either packaged or as a bulk item. Only buy what you really need with maybe a bit extra. You don't want it to go rancid.

- ✔ **Where to store it:** Store quinoa in a glass container in a dark cupboard. It lasts for approximately six months.

Always wash quinoa well to remove the bitter coating called *saponin*. Add water to a bowl to just cover the quinoa and lightly scrub the seeds for about 10 seconds. Strain and rinse in a strainer until the water runs clear.

Nutritional yeast

Nutritional yeast is made from a single-celled organism, which is grown on molasses and then harvested, washed, and dried with heat to kill or "deactivate" it. Because it's inactive, it doesn't froth or grow like baking yeast does; it has no leavening ability. It is yellowish and flaky and often comes sealed in a bag or container.

It adds flavor that can be described as cheesy, nutty, and savory. It can be added to soups, bean salads, and other dishes to enhance the taste, and it makes a great gravy.

✔ **Benefits:** Nutritional yeast is an excellent source of B vitamins, except B12 (unless you choose an enriched variety). It's packed with folic acid, selenium, zinc, and protein, and it contains no added sugars or preservatives.

✔ **Where to find it:** You can find nutritional yeast in the dry-goods or specialty-goods section of your local health-food or grocery store. Sometimes it can even be found in the vitamin and supplements aisle or in the refrigerator section. You only need one bag or container at a time, as you typically use this ingredient in small amounts.

✔ **Where to store it:** After the package is opened, it's best to keep it in a glass container in your fridge.

Miso

Miso is a fermented paste made from soy beans, a koji inoculant (bacteria), salt, and a grain (rice or barley). Just as grapes can be fermented into many different types of wine, soybeans can be fermented into many different flavors of miso. Miso is a concentrated food source and is rich in the eight essential amino acids — a staple of any healthy diet. Depending on the kind of miso, it can contain 12 percent to 20 percent protein. It's low in fat but high in salt, and therefore it should be used in moderation. Miso can be a substitute for Worcestershire sauce, salt, soy sauce, and other similar seasoning agents. It's typically used in soups, sauces, dressings, and even desserts.

✔ **Benefits:** Miso is an anti-carcinogen and is very effective in reducing the outcome of radiation, smoking, air pollution, and other environmental toxins. The darker the color of miso, the more potent its medicinal properties are.

✔ **Where to find it:** You'll find miso paste at most grocery stores; however, I recommend buying it at a health-food store, as it's likely to be a cleaner, organic version. It's found in the refrigerated section.

Always buy miso that is in a glass jar or container; the bagged versions are just messy. Then you can safely store it in your fridge for months. It's fermented, so it lasts a long time.

✔ **Where to store it:** If kept in an airtight glass container, refrigerated miso lasts a year or more.

Don't boil or overcook miso, as that destroys its beneficial microorganisms. Instead, just add it to warm water and stir until it dissolves. See the Chunky Miso Soup Recipe in Chapter 11.

What's the deal with fermenting?

Essentially, fermenting means converting the carbohydrates in foods into alcohol (not the kind that gets you drunk!). Examples of fermented foods are sauerkraut, kimchi, vinegar, tempeh, miso, yogurt, water kefir, and pickles, just to name a few. So why are these foods important?

Fermented foods have a lot of health benefits. They're rich in enzymes, which help digestion and absorption occur a lot more quickly. They're also rich in good bacteria, specifically lactobacillus acidophilus, which is an extremely beneficial flora found in the gut. By consuming healthy bacteria, such as the ones found in fermented foods, you can actually restore and re-balance the flora in your gut. This can lead to better vitamin and nutrient absorption. On a side note, fermented foods have a long shelf life without containing harmful preservatives, so you can enjoy your food longer without spoilage.

I go into much more detail about fermenting in my other book, *Fermenting For Dummies*, so pick up a copy if you want to know more about this world or even try your hand at your own fermenting!

Mushrooms

Mushrooms are the fruit of fungus and are among the most medicinal of all foods. They're different from other vegetables in that they don't convert sunlight to food. These fungi thrive on other organic matter and are often found growing on decaying wood. I know that doesn't sound appetizing, but if you're a mushroom eater already, you know that they're delicious!

- ✔ **Benefits:** Mushrooms are very effective at detoxification. In nature, they draw upon decaying matter, and in humans they're said to absorb and safely eliminate toxins. These toxins can include undesirable fats in the blood, pathogens, and excessive mucous in the respiratory system. Mushrooms are high in protein and are a good source of vitamin B2 and zinc.

    Mushrooms can be used in sauces, soups, stir-fries, salads, and stuffing. They soak up the essence of whatever they're cooked in, and the more finely they're cut, the more flavors they absorb.

    Before use, clean fresh mushrooms with a damp cloth. Also, dehydrating mushrooms intensifies their flavors, and they can be rehydrated with water.

- ✔ **Where to find them:** Mushrooms can be found at your local health-food store, grocery store, and farmers' markets. Buy only the fresh mushrooms you need, as they don't last that long — or try dried versions. You can discover many varieties of mushrooms to try. My favorites are portobello, porcini, cremini, shiitake, and button.

✓ **Where to store them:** Mushrooms can be safely stored in a brown paper bag in your fridge for up to a week. Make sure dried varieties are in a sealed container or glass jar for long-term storage.

Don't consume wild foraged mushrooms unless you're positive of their identity. Several varieties are lethal. Also, some commonly available mushrooms, such as white button mushrooms, portobellos, shiitakes, and creminis, contain small amounts of a compound that can be carcinogenic in extremely high doses. However, it's destroyed in cooking, so you needn't worry as long as you cook your mushrooms. Mushrooms taste better when you cook them, anyway.

Plant-based protein powders

A variety of powders are derived from key plant-based foods and have a high protein content. For the most part, they've been extracted, sprouted, or germinated to an optimal state for consumption. Many of these proteins are put out by commercial organic brands. Try your best to avoid anything that has been heat treated; look instead for raw or sprouted versions of pea or brown-rice proteins. You can buy containers of protein powder at health-food stores and even some grocery stores, and many online stores sell quality protein powders.

Pea protein

Peas are a member of the legume family. Legumes generally have an excellent nutritional profile: They're high in fiber, protein, and many vitamins and minerals and are a particularly exceptional source of amino acids. They are also rich in B vitamins and potassium. Because of peas' superior amino-acid profile, pea protein concentrates and isolates are a great plant-based option for those who have soy allergies.

Peas strengthen the kidneys and adrenal glands and therefore promote physical growth and development. Just like the protein in meat, peas promote the development of muscle mass, but unlike meat they don't add cholesterol, saturated fat, or toxic nitrogen byproducts.

Pea protein is especially great in smoothies and energy bars.

Brown-rice protein

Rice is one of the most consumed foods in the world by volume. Because rice has been unaltered over the years, the possibility of it causing an allergic reaction is low. Brown rice has a mild, nutty flavor and is less processed than white rice, making it nutritionally superior.

Because only its outermost layer (the hull) is removed, brown rice retains its nutritional value. Brown rice is high in manganese and contains large amounts of selenium, magnesium, and B vitamins. It's easy to digest and doesn't contain any soy for those who are allergic.

You can buy it in powder form — a good brown-rice powder should not have any additives or fillers. Its most common use is in smoothies.

Seeds

Seeds make up another important food group in a plant-based diet — and they're probably much more powerful and versatile than you think! You can find these seeds at health-food stores, grocery stores, and small specialty markets, as well as online. Here are a few you should stock:

Chia

Chia is a seed that is a member of the sage family. It looks like a flattened and washed-out poppy seed. Chia seeds are valued as an endurance food, especially among Native Americans. Chia seeds are second to flaxseeds in the line of highest sources of omega-3 fatty acids. The darker seeds are more nutritional compared to the gold variety. When chia seeds are soaked, they become highly mucilaginous (slimy). Eating them in this state lubricates dryness, relieves constipation, reduces nervousness, treats insomnia, and improves mental focus.

Chia seeds can be added to smoothies or juices and can create a gelatinous beverage. Add dry seeds ground or whole to granola, flours, or even in place of poppy seeds as a garnish.

Pumpkin

You're probably pretty familiar with what pumpkin seeds look like, but did you know they're higher in protein than most other seeds or nuts (29 percent protein) and are a valuable source of the essential omega-3 fatty acids? They're also rich in vitamins and minerals, including iron, zinc, phosphorus, vitamin A, calcium, and B vitamins. Pumpkin seeds are used for pinworms and intestinal parasites and are considered medicinal for the liver, colon, spleen, and pancreas.

They're available roasted or raw. As many of us can attest to at Halloween, light roasting improves their flavor and digestibility.

Season pumpkin seeds with sea salt or herbs of your choice. Spread seeds in a pan and roast in a preheated 300-degree oven for 15 minutes or until lightly toasted. Be careful not to over-bake!

Sunflower

Sunflower seeds are a daisy relative; both were cultivated by Native Americans. The shells can be black, white, brown, or black with white stripes. They're an energy tonic and a nurturing food used to treat constipation. Sunflower seeds contain more protein than beef and are 20 percent fat (mostly unsaturated). They're a good source of calcium; phosphorus; iron; vitamins A, D, and E; and several Bs.

Shelled sunflower seeds may substitute for nuts in many recipes. The seeds may be ground to a butter that is very similar to peanut butter. Whole seeds have a good shelf life, but if hulled they need to be refrigerated. Avoid discolored or rubbery seeds.

Hemp

Hempseeds come straight from the plant and are eaten raw, or commonly ground into powder. They're rich in omega-3 and omega-6 fatty acids. Hemp is a complete protein, containing all the essential amino acids, which boost the immune system and speed up recovery. Hemp is also a natural anti-inflammatory, which is a key factor in speeding up the repair of soft tissue damage caused by physical stress or exercise. Raw hemp products maintain their natural high levels of vitamins, minerals, high-quality balanced fats, antioxidants, fiber, and alkaline chlorophyll. Hemp protein is the easiest protein to digest and is instrumental in muscle tissue regeneration and metabolism.

It's great mixed into smoothies or granola or sprinkled on oatmeal, and you can make energy bars out of it — or just eat it raw, straight up.

Rounding Out the Rest of Your Goods

The following sections suggest other items to add to your grocery list, depending on the season and your tastes. The preceding section gives you the essentials, so use these lists to fill in the rest of your fridge and cupboards (and stomach).

Fresh produce

This is what you're going to find yourself buying most frequently, as you're going to want it fresh — meaning you have to purchase it in small quantities. Depending on where you find it, you can get produce pretty inexpensively, although you may have to do some shopping around.

Keep this basic produce on hand as much as possible, as it's so nutritious and versatile:

- Avocado
- Broccoli
- Cauliflower
- Fresh fruit (in season), such as bananas, apples, pears, kiwi, grapes, cherries, pineapple, and melons
- Leafy green vegetables, such as broccoli, kale, bok choy, cabbage, lettuce, and spinach
- Garlic
- Lemons and limes
- Mushrooms
- Onions (red and white)
- Sweet potatoes or squash
- Tomatoes

When you stash those items in your fridge, leave room for the following items. You'll likely buy these items less frequently, so be on the lookout for expiration dates:

- Fresh ginger
- Olives and pickles
- Sauerkraut
- Soy foods: miso paste, barley miso, tofu, and tempeh
- Yogurt from coconut milk, or coconut kefir

Frozen foods

Having some convenience foods and treats on hand is a great way to stay on track with your plant-based meals. This may mean all the difference between staying on and falling off the plant wagon — especially on those days when you're feeling a bit tired or unmotivated. Just use them in moderation, because things like frozen vegetables are truly *only* for the sake of convenience. Try to buy fresh whenever possible. Here's a list of frozen goods to get you started:

- Frozen berries, peaches, and mangos
- Frozen organic vegetables, including broccoli, edamame, peas, and spinach

✔ Non-dairy ice cream made from coconut or rice

✔ Sprouted-grain breads and wraps

✔ Tempeh

✔ Veggie burgers made from grains, nuts, and seeds

Note: In some cases, frozen vegetables and fruits are more nutritious than fresh vegetables, especially if the frozen versions are organic. They're often picked at peak ripeness and flash frozen soon afterward, thereby maintaining their nutrients. The nutrient content of fresh produce is affected by how much time passes between picking and eating, as nutrients degrade over time.

Staples to store in your pantry

Always keep these foundational items stocked in your pantry, cupboards, and the like. Some of these foods have a short shelf life, but you can keep others around for longer periods of time.

Goods with a shorter shelf life: Pastas, milks, and more

Make sure you buy these items in small amounts, and rotate your inventory frequently:

✔ **Baking goods:** Baking powder, baking soda, and vanilla (and other) extracts

✔ **Dried beans:** Black beans, chickpeas, kidney beans, lentils, pinto beans, and white beans

✔ **Egg replacements:** Ground flaxseeds or ground chia seeds

✔ **Flavorings:** Carob, cacao powder, sea salt, and wasabi powder

✔ **Flours:** Buckwheat flour, brown-rice flour, oat flour, kamut flour, or spelt flour

✔ **Herbs and spices:** Allspice, basil, bay leaves, chili powder, cinnamon, cloves, cumin, curry powder, five spice powder, garlic powder, ground ginger, ground mustard, marjoram, onion powder, oregano, paprika, rosemary, sage, thyme, turmeric, whole black pepper, and whole nutmeg

Store your herbs and spices away from heat and light sources. (In other words, don't store them over the oven or in the window, because the heat and light cause them to lose their flavor more quickly.) Replace herbs and spices that are older than one year. You can substitute one teaspoon of dried herbs for one tablespoon of chopped fresh herbs.

✔ **Milks:** Almond, carob, hempseed, oat, or chocolate or vanilla rice (store in the fridge after opening)

✔ **Natural sweeteners:** Coconut nectar; blackstrap molasses; brown-rice syrup; maple syrup; or whole, unrefined cane sugar

- ✔ **Nuts and seeds:** Almonds, cashews, pecans, popcorn kernels, pumpkin seeds, sesame seeds, shelled sunflower seeds, and walnuts

- ✔ **Pasta and noodles (whole grain):** Buckwheat soba noodles, spelt, kamut noodles, and brown-rice noodles

- ✔ **Pseudo grains:** Amaranth, buckwheat, quinoa, and wild rice

- ✔ **Sea vegetables:** Arame, dulse, hijiki, kombu, nori, and wakame

- ✔ **Teas:** Green, rooibos, and herbal

- ✔ **Thickeners:** Agar, arrowroot, and kudzu

- ✔ **Unsweetened dried fruit:** Apricots, cranberries, dates, figs, and raisins

- ✔ **Whole grains:** Barley, brown rice, millet, and spelt

- ✔ **Whole-grain products or sprouted grains:** Cereals, breads, pita breads, and wraps

Foods with longer shelf lives: Canned goods and condiments

Although these items have a long shelf life and make cooking and eating convenient, I recommend getting them only when necessary:

- ✔ Canned, BPA-free, organic tomatoes in diced, crushed, pate, or whole form

- ✔ Dijon mustard

- ✔ Unsweetened fruit jams (strawberry, blackberry, or raspberry) and apple butter

- ✔ Naturally brewed soy sauce, such as liquid amino acids, shoyu, and tamari (wheat free)

- ✔ Naturally sweetened ketchup — sweetened with agave or coconut nectar, which is much better than high-fructose corn syrup

- ✔ Nut and seed butters, such as almond, cashew, walnut, and tahini

- ✔ Oils, including olive, flaxseed, coconut, grapeseed, and toasted sesame

- ✔ Pineapple, mango, or yam puree (not ideal, but may be required in some baking)

- ✔ Salsa

- ✔ Tomato sauce

- ✔ Unsweetened coconut milk

- ✔ Vinegars, such as balsamic, brown rice, coconut, red wine, and unpasteurized apple cider

Getting the Must-Have Equipment

Having your kitchen set up correctly is just another way to make it easy and enjoyable to stay on track with your new plant-based habits. If everything you need is within arm's reach, it's easy to not only make delicious meals but also choose healthy snacks.

You want to have a few essential things on hand when it comes time to make all this delicious food. If you don't have the right tools, it's that much more difficult to cook. In the following sections, I outline some of the basics. Check off the ones you have, go shopping for others, and put the rest on your wish list.

I highly recommend investing in good cookware and bakeware up front. It may be pricey, but it's a true investment that really makes a difference. Your food is only as good as what it comes in contact with. Choose good-quality stainless steel whenever and wherever possible.

Handy utensils

You may be surprised by how many of these you already have at home. Some you may use, and some may still be wrapped up in a box because you don't know what to do with them! Here is a list of the basic utensils you want to make sure you have:

- ✔ **Bakeware:** You need a cookie sheet, muffin tray, glass baking dish, cake pan, and pie pan.

- ✔ **Colander:** This is similar to a strainer but has wider holes and a bigger base. This is good for washing vegetables and draining pasta.

- ✔ **Cutting boards (wooden):** You want at least one, maybe two, for cutting all your veggies. Aim for one that is at least 12 inches by 14 inches. You can get ones with rubber stoppers on the corners, or you can put a damp cloth beneath the board to prevent it from sliding.

- ✔ **Grater:** Use this for shredding vegetables.

- ✔ **Kitchen tongs:** Tongs are great for tossing stir-fries, mixing veggie salads, or picking up slices of tofu out of a pan. They're also good for plating food.

- ✔ **Knives:** Get yourself a set of good knives. If you're intimidated by the whole set, just start with these three: a serrated knife, a chef's knife, and a paring knife. See Figure 7-1 to see what they look like.

✔ **Measuring cups:** Get yourself a dry set of measuring cups for grains, flours, and seeds and wet measuring cups for rice milk, maple syrup, olive oil, and the like — opt for the ones where you can see the measurements looking down.

✔ **Measuring spoons:** Get a set — preferably stainless steel — with measurements for 1 tablespoon, 1 teaspoon, ½ teaspoon, ¼ teaspoon, and ⅛ teaspoon.

✔ **Microplane:** This type of grater is great for zesting lemons and oranges or grating ginger or garlic.

✔ **Mixing bowls (stainless steel):** These are lightweight and easy to clean. Glass bowls are also nice and clean up very well.

✔ **Pots and pans:** You want to have a range of sizes, including a small saucepan, a sauté pan, a skillet, and a soup pot.

Chemically coated pans can leach harmful chemicals and toxins into your food and into your body. Non-stick means toxic!

✔ **Spatula (metal):** This is essential for making perfect pancakes or flipping items in a pan.

✔ **Spoons (wooden and stainless steel):** You want a variety of spoons for mixing, stirring, and moving food around in a pan. Get a variety that feel and look nice and that clean up well.

✔ **Steaming basket or insert:** It's great to have a steamer on hand for quick veggie prep.

✔ **Strainer:** Preferably you'll get a fine mesh, bowl-shaped one. This is a handy tool for washing grains, nuts, and seeds. You want the mesh to be fine enough that things like quinoa and amaranth don't seep through.

✔ **Vegetable peeler:** Be sure to get one with a good hand grip and a wide blade. You want a peeler that will do a variety of veggies and fruits, from carrots and squashes to apples.

✔ **Wire whisk:** This is great for combining liquids, such as a salad dressing, or mixing wet ingredients into dry ones.

Figure 7-1:
If you don't want to buy a full knife set, start with these three basics.

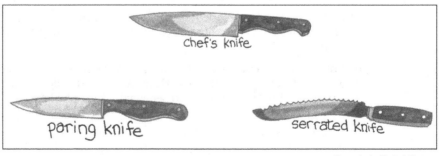

Illustration by Elizabeth Kurtzman

Glass versus plastic storage

When storing food, you should always use glass containers. Although plastic is cheaper and lighter, plastic is just downright harmful to your health, as it leaches toxins into anything that is stored in it. This goes for solid foods and liquids, no matter whether you store things in a cupboard, in the fridge, or in the freezer.

You also most certainly *do not* want to put plastic in the microwave. In my opinion, you should just try to rid yourself of plastic altogether. Glass is not only cleaner and lasts longer, but it generally just looks better overall.

I encourage you to become conscious about the environment and your health all in one. You have a choice to make every day when it comes to food, including where you get it, how you take it home, and how you store it.

Non-essential (but helpful) appliances

Here are some other fun and helpful pieces of equipment that make your kitchen time and cooking experiences that much more efficient:

- ✔ **Countertop blender:** You most definitely want one of these. This is essential for smoothies, cold soups, and even "ice cream."
- ✔ **Food processor:** This appliance is fabulous for quickly chopping, grating, and mixing larger quantities of ingredients.
- ✔ **Funnel:** This is good for pouring soups, sauces, purees, and other liquids into smaller jars.
- ✔ **Immersion blender:** This is a fabulous and handy tool for blending soups right in the pot. It's also good for sauces and dressings.
- ✔ **Mortar and pestle:** You're going to have fun with this one grinding your own herbs and spices.
- ✔ **Toaster oven:** This is a handy device so you don't have to turn on your regular oven when you just want to warm up something small.

Microwave days are over

Get rid of your microwave! This may sound daunting and even threatening, as this convenient, easy-to-use appliance has been one of the most purchased and widely used in the last few decades. However, microwaves emit electromagnetic waves (radiation) into your food, which changes the molecular structure of the food. It's not a whole food anymore! You then ingest it, which can't be good for your cells or your body.

A microwave may seem like a simple solution to get something hot quickly, but it's just as easy to reheat or warm up your food on the stove top or in a toaster oven — it may take longer, but you may live longer!

Finding Alternatives to Common Ingredients

In Chapter 6, I mention that you can swap out plant-based ingredients for some of your favorite and most comforting ingredients. You may be at a loss and wonder how it's even possible to find a plant-based alternative to certain foods. The following sections cover some common ingredients and what the main go-tos are in the veggie world.

Milk

Luckily you can find a plethora of non-dairy milk alternatives, which are available at stores or easy enough to make at home. Some varieties include almond, rice, hempseed, coconut, cashew, and Brazil-nut milk. You can easily substitute these (in equal measurement) into any recipe that calls for milk.

Choosing alternative milk doesn't mean you're missing out on calcium. Many nutritious plant-based foods, such as almonds, kale, and bok choy, are loaded with these nutrients. They're not just found in milk!

Eggs

People are often nervous about how to substitute an egg. "I mean, what's going to give that muffin its 'stock' if there isn't an egg?" you may be worrying. Well, you have more options than you likely think you do!

Try these; each makes the equivalent of one egg:

- Three tablespoons of ground flaxseeds or ground chia seeds plus six tablespoons of water (soak for five to ten minutes to allow the mixture to become gelatinous)
- ¼ cup pureed banana
- ¼ cup apple sauce

Meat

Meat is out on a plant-based diet. For a hearty, rich texture and something that fills you up, the main plant-based items to stock up on are tempeh, tofu, beans, and portobello mushrooms. Each of these items has a hearty, chewy texture, and you can marinate them in pretty much any sauce. You can also chop them up, grind them up, or use them any way you would use meat: as burgers, in stews and chili, or just baked on your plate.

Cheese

This is usually one of the most difficult items for people to give up. Most people are addicted to cheese. The good news is that the plant world offers creamy, soft textures that are rich and decadent and can be used in place of cheese. Here are some of my favorites: sliced avocado, soaked and blended cashews, sprouted soft organic tofu, and nutritional yeast. All of these can be added to pizza, quesadillas, tacos, sandwiches, and other dishes that need a "cheesy" flavor.

As for store-bought cheese, the Daiya brand is becoming quite popular in homes and restaurants, as it's the closest thing to cheese that the plant-based world has been able to come up with so far. The other benefit is that it's not soy-based. (Most non-dairy cheeses are overly processed versions of soy, which can be harmful to your health.) It's still technically a packaged food, so keep your consumption to a minimum (such as during those times when you have a serious craving, and nothing else will do).

Avoid soy cheeses and rice cheeses, as they're extremely processed and don't quite hit the spot. Also, these options sometimes contain trace amounts of dairy.

If you find it really hard to give up cow dairy, just know that choosing sheep-milk and goat-milk cheeses can be an option as you're transitioning. They're lower in lactose and easier to digest, and from an ethical standpoint sheep and goats are treated much better than cows in the food industry.

Thickeners

Ever wonder what holds your meat gravy together? You probably don't want to know. Even cornstarch, which is plant-based, isn't good for you because it's likely genetically modified. So go for arrowroot powder, kudzu, or tapioca. Each of these items makes your sauces and puddings gooey from natural sources.

You can find these items in most health-food stores or grocery stores in the baking section.

Mock meats

Textured vegetable protein (TVP) is a byproduct of soybean oil and is used as a fake meat. You can find all sorts of "meatless meats" out there right now. Although they're technically plant-based because they don't have animal products in them, they are processed foods with loads of additives and aren't something I recommend when you need a meaty fix. Don't eat the mock versions of foods; stick with the meat alternatives I mention earlier.

Chapter 8

Being a Savvy Shopper

*W*hen you embark on a new diet, it can be hard to figure out what's what and where to buy different items (heck, even if you've been eating plant-based for a while, you may still be stumped when it comes to procuring the best stuff). Navigating farmers' markets, health-food stores, and the organic section in your neighborhood grocery store can be enough to make you feel like you're running in circles.

Luckily, I have a few general rules that you can use to navigate toward the healthy and away from the traps. In this chapter, I go into these tips in detail: Shop the perimeter of the grocery store (where the fresh foods are stocked), avoid the center aisles (where junk food and sugared cereals lurk), choose real foods (such as 100 percent fruit juice or 100 percent whole grain), stay clear of foods with cartoons on the label, and avoid foods that contain more than five ingredients or artificial ingredients that you can't pronounce.

I also suggest other places to shop for plant-based foods, and I explain what the terms *organic* and *GMO* mean and why you should be familiar with them.

Reading Product Labels

Before purchasing something, you have to decide what you want to spend your money on. As a conscientious plant-based consumer, it's your duty to look into everything you buy and eat. Obviously I advocate a diet that is high in whole foods and low in packaging; however, sometimes you just can't avoid packaged foods, so you need to be able to sift and sort through what's good and what's not so good. And what better place to start than with the label? Here are some quick tips to get you started on being a label-reading ninja.

Analyzing the ingredients, not the numbers

I'm not a fan of counting. I'm most interested in the ingredients of a food, not the calories. Generally speaking, *what* the product is made up of is much more important than the grams of protein and fat. Knowing *where* those grams come from is what actually makes a difference in your body.

You need to reference only two numbers, and those are the listed amounts of sugar and fiber. In a second, I go into more specifics, but remember that those numbers are just guidelines to help you gauge how nutritious the food is. This may be hard to adjust to at first, as we have become a society that is . . . let's see, how to put this delicately . . . *obsessed* with the amount of protein, carbs, and fat in a serving. But trust me, this becomes less important to you when you start to understand that "low fat" or "low carb" isn't all that good for you after all (more on that later in this chapter).

When you look at the nutrition label, here's what you're looking for:

- ✓ **The order of ingredients:** The ingredients are listed in order of prevalence, with the most prevalent coming first. See which ingredients are listed in which order. Of particular note is the first ingredient: Is it something bad, like high-fructose corn syrup, or is it healthy, like whole grain? If you see any "bad" ingredients listed, make sure they're as close to the end of the list as possible (flip back to Chapter 3 for a refresher on the good guys and the bad guys).

  If the first three ingredients aren't whole, recognizable items, don't buy the product.

- ✓ **The amount and type of sugar:** When it comes to sugar, you first want to see how much is in the food (ideally not much more than 5 to 10 grams per serving, depending on the item and the grams overall). Next you need to identify the source of that sugar. Select products that have healthier sources (such as maple syrup, coconut nectar, or agave — more on sweeteners in Chapters 3 and 13). Knowing what the sugar is made up of can make all the difference.

- ✓ **The amount of fiber:** Depending on what the product is, it's likely to have some form of fiber (especially because it's plant-based). Look for items that have more than five grams of fiber per serving. High-fiber foods are more wholesome and better for your digestion and overall health. (See Chapter 3 for more on fiber.)

Understanding common terms

Unfortunately, most of us have been misled for years by corporations marketing their food products. We mistakenly rely on food labels for an accurate picture of the nutritional value of the foods we consume. Phrases like "all natural," "made from whole grain," and "lowfat" seem like they describe healthy foods. Well, that's not always true; you have to look a little closer and be a detective when it comes to food labels. For starters, if you want to achieve a healthier lifestyle, be skeptical of the following misleading terms:

- ✔ **All natural:** This is a widely used term in food labeling and marketing and has a variety of definitions, most of which are vague. The term is designed to make you assume that these foods have been minimally processed and don't contain manufactured ingredients. However, the lack of standards in most jurisdictions means that the term assures nothing at all. In some countries, the term *natural* is defined and enforced; however, in North America, it has no regulated meaning. Sometimes folks think *all natural* is synonymous with *organic*. The term organic, however, actually has a stricter legal definition in most countries that is usually paired with an additional international standard.

- ✔ **Low calorie:** When a product is diminished of its calories, chemical ingredients are often used to lighten up the product. These may be in the form of aspartame or other additives. Overall, consuming too few calories leaves you feeling grumpy, weak, tired, and ineffective during your workday and your workouts. The other thing to remember is that most food calories come from fat and carbohydrates, so it's more about where those fats and carbohydrates are coming from, not necessarily how much of them you're eating.

The skinny on "low carb" and "carb free"

These terms became ever so popular during the craze of high-protein, low-carb fad diets. But look where that has gotten us: Most people go on a low-carb diet for weight loss and nothing else. With that singular goal, dieters typically don't focus on overall health, and often these individuals end up gaining their weight back.

When carbs are lowered or taken out, your body needs you to replace them with something, which can lead to consuming more fat, protein, or sometimes even sugar substitutes (which, in turn, just make you crave more sugar). Depriving your body of carbs leads you to crave sugar sooner or later. So go ahead and eat those carbs — just stick to complex carbohydrate sources, such as brown rice, sweet potatoes, oats, and fresh fruit.

✔ **Lowfat or fat free:** Remember, your body needs certain fats to function properly. When you remove fat from your diet, usually you consume more sugar to compensate for the nutrients your body is craving. This defeats your purpose because too much sugar consumption can increase your caloric intake and contribute to weight gain, whereas good, healthy fats won't unless you eat them in excess (see Chapter 3 for a refresher on good fats).

✔ **Made from whole grain:** This is a phrase you want to look out for when you buy bread products or anything with grains in it. Just because something is "whole grain" doesn't mean it's the real deal. Unfortunately, a lot of products get away with making this claim because the manufacturer uses whole grain somewhere (in small quantity) in the product, but the rest of the ingredient list is usually processed or refined flours. Unless the label says 100 percent whole grain, you have no idea how much (or how little) whole grain and fiber you're truly getting.

The gluten-free craze

For a growing number of people, maintaining a diet free of gluten is a necessary way of life because of celiac disease (a chronic condition in which the body is unable to break down gluten). However, eating a gluten-free diet has become trendy even for those without celiac disease.

It's important to address your reasons for eating gluten free. Are you sensitive to gluten, or do you just believe that you'll be "healthier" if you go gluten free? The craze is a problem because the gluten-free label is now overused on products that are naturally gluten free. Not to mention, gluten-free foods aren't automatically healthy; some are made with processed or poor ingredients, such as canola oil, sugar, potato starch, and cornstarch, among other additives. Eating these processed foods is a common mistake that people make when going gluten free.

Also, note that some gluten-free items contain traces of milk, butter, or eggs (used as a gluten replacement to restore a soft texture),

so as a plant-based eater, you want to double check the ingredient list. Many whole foods are naturally gluten free, and these should be the main part of your diet regardless of your level of gluten sensitivity.

Remember: Many people who are sensitive to processed wheat products (but don't have celiac disease) can still eat less-processed forms of wheat, such as spelt and kamut, and other gluten-containing grains, such as barley and rye. They may feel a lot better, especially if the grains are sprouted (see Chapter 3). And don't forget the many wonderful gluten-free grains, such as quinoa, brown rice, millet, and teff.

The point is, don't avoid a food before knowing what you're doing and why you're doing it. However, if it makes you feel better to eat gluten free, then by all means proceed in the most healthy and wholesome way possible.

✔ **Sugar free:** Something that's labeled sugar free probably contains artificial sweeteners instead. If you think that artificial sweeteners are better options than sugar, you're setting yourself up for disaster. Chemical sweeteners like aspartame trick your body into thinking it's getting sugar when it's not and actually make you crave more (real) sugar. Stay natural and choose products that contain sweeteners like dates, date paste, date sugar, honey, maple syrup, and coconut sugar.

Reading the hidden ingredient list

Some ingredients you actually see on a food label, and some you don't — either because they're masked by other ingredients or because they're listed as names the average consumer may not recognize. To help you decipher this seemingly foreign language, here are some of the main hidden (and not-so-hidden) bad guys to watch for:

✔ **BHA:** A preservative used in breakfast cereals. Vague research suggests that it is carcinogenic.

✔ **Parabens:** These are synthetic preservatives that inhibit mold and yeast in food. The problem is that parabens can disrupt your body's hormonal balance.

✔ **Partially hydrogenated oils:** These trans fats can pose a threat to your arteries.

✔ **Caramel coloring:** The name makes it sound like a relatively natural formula of water and sugar, but the food industry adds ammonia, which is carcinogenic. Most often, this is found in dark sodas, but it can also show up in whole-grain breads and crackers.

✔ **Castoreum:** This is a flavor enhancer. It may not sound that harmful, but it's animal-derived. (Are you ready for this? It's a secretion from the castor gland, which is located near the anus of mature beavers.) This ingredient is often listed as raspberry or vanilla flavoring.

✔ **Hydrolyzed vegetable protein:** Even though this is a plant protein, it's derived from chemically broken down amino acids. This process forms glutamate. When this glutamate finds free sodium in your body, it becomes MSG (a salt commonly used as a flavor enhancer that is tied to adverse reactions). So, in essence, hydrolyzed vegetable protein is an additive that can cause the same reactions as MSG: headaches, nausea, and bloating.

✔ **Sugars such as fructose, sucrose, and dextrose:** Don't be fooled by the different terms; these all act the same in the body. Look out for and avoid products with these ingredients on the label.

Conquering the Grocery Store

You've got your list, and you know *what* to look for. Now let's get into the *where* of it all. Although you can use non-grocery-store resources (I talk about those in the next section), most people are probably most familiar with a standard grocery store, so that's where I want to start. This section is all about helping you figure out how to navigate through the store so you can steer around the bad stuff and start filling your cart with the good stuff.

Picking up produce

When you first enter a grocery store, you more than likely find yourself right in the produce section, amongst all the colorful fruits and vegetables that you should fill your cart with. So go ahead — start your shopping trip out right there by grabbing your usuals — whatever you're most comfortable with already (maybe things like carrots, broccoli, and bananas).

Next, I encourage you to explore new terrain. Perhaps that means venturing over to that corner that's filled with lots of green bunches of leaves (it's okay if you're a little intimidated). Just get to know them — a lot of them look similar, but they are indeed different. Check the labels above and below them and get used to noticing what kale, collards, Swiss chard, and dandelion look like. Compare their colors, leaf shapes and sizes, and stems. Each of them holds different possibilities for you. These will become your new friends as you start to round out your plant-based diet.

If you're feeling a little lost, don't be afraid to ask a grocery worker for help. They know a lot about what each piece of produce is, what it does, and how to cook it.

Also on the labels, you may notice a note about where the items come from. Now, this is the tricky (and sometimes unfortunate, depending on where you live) part, as you want to buy items that are grown close to where you live — ideally within the same country. If you live far from where fresh produce grows, at least aim for items that are closest. You can only do the best you can with where you are. I'm guilty of being a consumer of avocados, bananas, and mangos, which are most definitely not local to where I live!

Finally, when it comes to choosing organic versus local produce, just use your best judgment. To help you, the Environmental Working Group, an organization that provides information to protect public health and the environment, has done a fabulous job of outlining two lists, called the Dirty Dozen and the Clean Fifteen. They help consumers determine the best, safest produce to buy.

✔ **The Dirty Dozen Plus:** This list started with 12 items but has increased to 14. These types of produce are the biggest carriers of pesticides and chemical residues that can harm your health. When you buy these foods, you want to buy them in organic form and not in conventionally grown versions (as much as possible). If you do buy them conventionally once in a while, be sure to wash them well.

- Apples
- Celery
- Cherry tomatoes
- Collard greens
- Cucumbers
- Grapes
- Kale
- Nectarines
- Peaches
- Peppers
- Potatoes
- Spinach
- Strawberries
- Summer squash

Chemical residues and pesticides don't only reside on skins and peels; they're embedded within most parts of the fruit or vegetable.

✔ **The Clean Fifteen:** On the other hand, this is the produce that's okay to eat conventionally (that is, it doesn't have to be organic) in moderation, as it carries the least amount of pesticides and chemical residues:

- Asparagus
- Avocados
- Cabbage
- Cantaloupe
- Eggplant
- Grapefruit
- Kiwi
- Mangos
- Mushrooms

- Onions
- Papaya
- Pineapples
- Sweet corn
- Sweet peas
- Sweet potatoes

Please note that these lists change from year to year. Keep up to date with the most current lists at www.ewg.org.

Steering clear of interior aisles

Most people do a lot of their shopping in the interior aisles of a grocery store because the rows upon rows of colorful boxes of packaged food are convenient and tend to feed our sodium and sugar addictions (not to mention, they appear to be cheaper, more filling, and longer lasting than fresh produce). However, you should do your best to fight the urge to cruise the interior aisles; instead, stay away from them as much as possible — they contain very few products that are good for you (I talk more about the "good" things in a second). Here are three reasons to avoid these aisles:

- ✔ **Packaged products have unnatural shelf lives:** The fact that something can sit on the shelf for a long time doesn't make it better. You may think that a long expiration date is good because it's more economical, but more time means more preservatives, which means more manmade chemicals have been added to the food. Many of these preservatives have been found to cause health problems ranging from headaches to full-blown skin rashes, so be wary of breads, crackers, and cookies that have an expiration date that's longer than six months.

- ✔ **A cheap price means cheap ingredients:** It may seem like a perk that you can get some items for less dough, but the cost comes in somewhere, and that is likely as the toll the foods take on your health. The only reason companies can get away with lower prices is that they're using cheaper ingredients, which makes for a poor-quality product and another good reason to avoid the interior aisles and the food in them.

- ✔ **Packaged products have layers of packaging:** This isn't just a nutritional reason but also an environmental one. Most packaging is just waste that ends up in our landfills, which of course has a negative impact on the Earth. Health-wise, the more packaging an item has, the less fresh it is. When a product has layers of packaging (such as an outer box, plus inner wrapping, and sometimes even more), it's a big red flag that the manufacturer had to use a number of resources just to keep that food synthetically fresh. If you can't avoid packaged foods altogether, do your best to at least choose products with minimal packaging.

Dipping into the interior aisles when you must

Of course sometimes you need to venture into the aisles to get certain packaged items. Although most of the products on the shelves are garbage for your health, you can still find some relatively wholesome options with no added ingredients or preservatives (or at least they're as minimal as possible).

Some of the healthier items to look for in the aisles include:

- ✔ Dry grains, such as quinoa, millet, rice, brown-rice pasta, and whole oats
- ✔ Non-dairy milks, such as rice milk or almond milk
- ✔ Whole-grain or brown-rice crackers made with wholesome ingredients
- ✔ Raw and plain nuts and seeds
- ✔ Dried organic legumes and beans (and even some canned organic beans)
- ✔ Snack foods like brown-rice cakes, organic tortilla chips, and salsa
- ✔ Liquids and sauces, such as tamari, tahini, olive oil, and apple-cider vinegar
- ✔ 100 percent fruit juices made from apple, pear, or lemon

Seeing what's lurking in the freezer

The freezer section of the grocery store can also be a scary place if you're not aware of what's contained within those cases. Nothing is wrong with freezing per se, as it keeps food in the state in which it was frozen. However, in many grocery stores, the freezer section acts just like the aisles, with rows upon rows of colorful, enduring packages filled with foods that have all kinds of unhealthy ingredients. Even many plant-based foods, such as veggie burgers, pizza, and frozen veggies, need to be considered very carefully, as you want to make sure that they're made up of quality ingredients that you recognize, with no traces of dairy or other animal products, and that they're organic and not genetically modified (see more on that later in this chapter).

Just because you choose a frozen food that is, say, all vegetables, that doesn't mean it's good for you. I recommend choosing these only in a pinch (or if it means that you wouldn't otherwise have any veggies at all). Some vegetables (preferably organic ones) are frozen at their peak, which means all of the nutrients are left somewhat intact, whereas conventional frozen veggies are likely to have fewer nutrients to begin with, and when they're frozen they lose even more. Not to mention, frozen veggies are less versatile. For example, you can't make a salad with frozen vegetables; they carry lots of water and are always soggy. That said, some are better than others.

Here are some of the healthier options you can find in your freezer section that are okay to take home:

- ✔ Fruits and berries
- ✔ Non-dairy coconut-based ice cream (in moderation for a treat)
- ✔ Organic veggie burgers made from beans, nuts, and seeds
- ✔ Sprouted-grain breads or wraps
- ✔ Tempeh
- ✔ Veggies like spinach, peas, butternut squash, and organic corn

Shopping Off the Beaten Path

When you're immersed in this world of plant-based eating for a bit of time, grocery-store shopping may begin to lose its appeal. You may find yourself wanting to set foot instead on alternative ground, which is actually now becoming more mainstream. Shopping at places like farmers' markets and health-food stores or getting involved with a local community-supported agriculture (CSA) service will likely become your new terrain for shopping. Why? First, the diversity of products that fall within your new plant-based standards are boundless in these locations (although you still have to be a discerning consumer, as organic cheeses and the like still aren't healthy snacks). Also, at places like farmers' markets, you get access to some of the freshest produce. Not to mention, when you shop at places like these, you support smaller businesses that typically have as much interest in your health as they do in making a sale. All around, you feel better about your choices. Let's take a look at why these places may be the next wave of your grocery-shopping experience.

Farmers' markets

Farmers' markets have popped up everywhere. They're a gathering of local vendors and farmers offering produce (and sometimes other fresh items) for direct sale to consumers. They usually happen weekly in a public place, such as a park or community center, and are typically busy. You won't find everything of a certain category in one place like you do at a grocery store. Every vendor has something different to offer.

The main benefit of farmers' markets, aside from all the food being extremely fresh, is that you get the chance to talk to the farmers about their products. They can tell you all about your new find, how to prepare it, and where exactly it came from. You can even ask about the growing methods, such as what pesticides were used (if any) and when it was harvested.

Community-supported agriculture (CSA) programs

This is a program in which consumers purchase annual or seasonal *shares* in farmers' land and receive fresh, seasonal produce from that farm in exchange for their monetary investment. In some cases, you pre-pay before the growing season. In other cases, you pay weekly for a delivery or pick up your share at a designated meeting place. These days, we're starting to see an evolution away from single-farm CSAs to multi-farm CSA services that give customers a wider variety of foods and more choices (which can sometimes be customized online). This is a nice way to get produce and sometimes other specialty goods without having to fight traffic in the parking lot (or aisles, for that matter).

CSAs are an especially helpful service to use when you're just starting out on a plant-based diet because the produce is sometimes selected for you (which can feel way less intimidating than trying to pick out your own stuff at the store). It's a great way to learn about different fruits and veggies and when they're at the height of their freshness. You can likely find CSAs in your area by doing an online search.

Health-food stores

Every major city — and most smaller ones — have at least a few health-food stores, and I'm not just talking about Whole Foods. You can typically find a whole slew of smaller, privately or family-run businesses that are committed to stocking good-quality products, clean packaged products, and nutritional supplements.

Health-food stores are typically much smaller than supermarkets, so it's much easier to find what you're looking for, which makes them convenient and easy places to stock up. You may also get to know the owners well, making it likely that they'll order things in for you by request or make other special arrangements with you if needed. Either way, shopping experiences at health-food stores are typically a lot smoother and more enjoyable than shopping at conventional grocery stores.

Just because you're in a health-food store doesn't mean that the staff are qualified to give nutritional advice or well-versed in the potential side effects of supplements. You need to be an educated consumer even in a health-food store.

Grow your own veggies, control your product from seed to mouth

Growing your own garden has so many benefits and is an amazing way to get fresh, organic vegetables and fruits into your body! Consider these five benefits of growing your own veggies:

✔ **High in nutrition:** Homegrown produce is likely organic produce, which means you're not using any pesticides or other contaminants. This means that the food can have a higher vitamin and mineral content than store-bought foods.

✔ **Fresh taste:** Foods that are free of pesticides and harvested straight from the garden are fresher and taste better.

✔ **Cost effective:** Growing your own vegetables significantly reduces your food costs. It also saves you time at the grocery store, giving you more time in your garden!

✔ **Environmentally friendly:** Home gardening lowers your carbon footprint by helping prevent soil erosion, improve water and air quality, save energy, and reduce transportation costs.

✔ **Fun, educational, and beautiful:** Gardening can be a fun and satisfying experiment for individuals, families, and children. It also helps create a beautiful personal space.

To figure out how to begin your garden, contact the farmers in your community, whether at farmers' markets or through searches online, or contact a local cooperative extension office. I'm sure many of them are willing to give you a little lesson on how to make the best use of your backyard. You can also try gardening clubs, community gardens, and even gardening exchanges (where people who have yard space but don't know what to do with it partner with experienced gardeners who come in and garden, splitting the produce 50-50). Even if you live in an apartment, you can get your green thumb on with potted plants and vertical gardening techniques.

Organic and GMO: Figuring Out What It All Means to a Plant-Based Diet

Lots of people these days are talking about what it means to eat organic. I know it's hard to make sense of, so I break it down once and for all. Incidentally, this also brings to light the label *GMO* (genetically modified organism), which is becoming a hot topic of discussion because of the prevalence of GMO foods and the health dangers they present.

Without screening your foods for and understanding these labels, you're doing your body and your health a disservice — especially if you're a new plant-based eater making all kinds of transitions to better your overall well-being. This is just one more step in the right direction of good health.

Is organic all it's cracked up to be?

Eating organic is all about making a choice to eat foods that aren't treated with pesticides, herbicides, fungicides, and the like. It also likely supports agricultural practices that preserve and work toward bettering the condition of the soil. Organic soil has more nutrients, including minerals. This makes for foods that all around taste better and are better for you. The standards for organic food come in several categories:

- **100 percent organic:** Contains *only* organic ingredients and must be produced without synthetic fertilizers, pesticides, antibiotics, genetic engineering, irradiation, or growth hormones. A U.S. Department of Agriculture (USDA) or Canadian seal of certification may appear on the product.

- **Organic:** Made with at least 95 percent organic ingredients. The remaining 5 percent must be approved by the USDA. No ionizing radiation is allowed. A USDA or Canadian seal may appear on the product.

- **Made with organic ingredients:** Made with at least 70 percent organic ingredients. The remaining 30 percent may be agricultural products that aren't produced according to organic standards. It must be clear which ingredients are organic. These products can't display the USDA or Canadian organic seal.

Many small organic farms can't afford the process of official certification, even though they adhere to all the organic practices the regulations require. You may encounter farms like this at your local farmers' market, so feel free to ask the farmers directly about whether they follow sustainable farming practices.

It's not always possible to stick to organic eating 100 percent, but as with anything else in this book, just do the best you can. Refer to the Dirty Dozen and Clean Fifteen lists I mention earlier in this chapter to help guide you when prioritizing your decisions about organic eating.

Local versus organic: Can you have it all?

When it comes to local, organic, or local and organic, people get confused and want to know which is better. From my perspective, if you can get your hands on both, that is generally the way to go — but not always.

When you have to make the choice between local non-organic or organic from across the world, it may be in your best interest to choose local. When food (even organic food) travels long distances, it loses its enzymes, nutrients, and life force, so you're left with an organic strawberry from South America that may have ripened on a truck, train, or plane. This means that unnatural gases and methods have been used to artificially stimulate the growth process.

In the end, you just need to do the best you can and make the best choices you can at a given time.

What's all this talk about GMOs?

A GMO is a genetically modified organism — sounds appetizing, right? You should know that most foods (that aren't labeled otherwise) contain genetically modified organisms. Sounds crazy, right? But GMOs can be found among crops such as soy, corn, and canola, and some fruits and vegetables you likely encounter daily. As a plant-a-tarian, you'd better watch out, as these ingredients are the basis of most commercial and packaged foods. A simple solution, of course, is to just stop eating these foods and instead eat whole foods that are organic. Sometimes it may not be that simple, but you've got to do the best you can. Luckily, governments across the globe are developing standards to help you identify which products contain GMOs.

Numerous scientific claims have created substantial debate about whether GMOs are beneficial to us. The initial theory was that GMOs could help prevent world hunger, give the world new varieties of foods, improve rural livelihoods, and help facilities and the environment. Instead, they have done more harm than good. GMOs have proven to be unsustainable, as farmers have to purchase new seeds every year while destroying the land (because GMO crops can encourage herbicide-resistant weeds and insecticide-resistant pests that infest non-GMO crops). GMOs have also created numerous allergies, especially to soy, and health problems, all while contaminating large sources of our food supply.

The original goals of GMOs aren't being accomplished. In fact, Europe has already figured this out, and many European countries ban most GMO crops. Unfortunately, North America hasn't picked up on this trend. Large companies that produce GMO seeds will do anything they can to protect their seeds and make sure that their seeds are the only ones used by a majority of North American farmers.

Although we're facing a sad truth, there is something you can do. You have a choice each time you buy food. Seek out resources like the Non-GMO Project, which helps consumers find products that are free of GMOs. It's important to know what you can do as a consumer and what you can do for your health. Check out www.nongmoproject.com for more information.

Chapter 9

Boosting Your Plant-Based Diet with Supplements

In This Chapter

▶ Grasping the role of supplements and using them properly on a plant-based diet

▶ Discovering the best forms of plant-based supplements and when to take them

*T*ypically, you should be able to get most if not all the nutrients you need from natural, organic whole foods; however, sometimes your health may require an additional boost. When it does, you can get that boost in the form of supplements. Supplements are doses of vitamins, minerals, fiber, amino acids, and other nutrients that you can take independently of food when they are necessary.

No matter your needs or health issues, a plant-based natural supplement may help improve your quality of life as you work toward getting healthier, leaner, and stronger. Supplements can be great things when used properly, but they can also cause problems if used incorrectly. This chapter goes through different plant-based supplements and how to use them to enhance your health and well-being.

Understanding the Basics of Supplements

The basic gist of supplements is that they help you stay healthy or beat sickness more quickly because they fortify your system. One thing I always like to say is that if you give your body the tools it needs to do the job properly, it self-corrects and protects your longevity and health. The average healthy individual who has a sensible, balanced diet and low-stress lifestyle doesn't necessarily need to take supplements regularly; however, there are times in a healthy person's life when certain supplements can be helpful on a daily, monthly, or yearly basis.

Here are a couple of other requirements I have for using supplements:

✔ Take them only for a short period of time as set out by a health practitioner.

✔ Take them *in conjunction with* a healthy, whole-food, plant-based diet and *not as a replacement for* a good diet, except in extreme cases (healing, traveling, or other special circumstances).

If you're considering using supplements, work with your health-care practitioner to figure out if you need to take them and, if you do, which ones you need.

Recognizing why you need supplements

You can find all sorts of reasons to need or want to take supplements. Used properly, they:

✔ Can help as a preventive approach to maintain or improve health (promote organ vitality and involvement).

✔ May be used in conjunction with a whole-foods, plant-based diet as the primary treatment or in support of other treatments for a variety of symptoms, short-term illnesses, and chronic diseases.

✔ Are increasingly used by nutritionists, physicians, and other health-care professionals as treatment for a multitude of problems.

✔ Can help with stress reduction and management.

✔ Can help people who are dieting ensure that they're getting the micronutrients required.

✔ Can help kids — who tend not to eat a balanced diet or who consume sugary foods — maintain proper levels of nutrients.

✔ Can help elderly people whose digestive systems aren't always working optimally and some whose nutrient needs have increased.

✔ Can help anyone who takes in a lot of sugar maintain proper levels of nutrients, because sugar is a nutrient-depleting substance devoid of its own nutrients.

✔ Can help provide smokers with additional support to battle the *free radicals* (unstable, irritating molecules) they harbor from inhaling smoke.

✔ Can help boost a system that's been run down by regular alcohol use, which depletes nutrients.

✔ Can help with carbohydrate metabolism and maintaining blood-sugar levels and with fat accumulation in the liver.

It's essential to take only the supplements you need, and only when you need them.

Getting to the bottom of multivitamins

One of the most common supplements is a multivitamin. But watch out — most multivitamins are completely synthetic. They're produced and processed with petroleum and crushed industrial rock or hydrogenated sugars. Tons of medical research has concluded that food nutrients are far superior to synthetics. One main reason they're insufficient is the complete lack of enzymes. Enzymes play a huge role in the utilization of nutrients and how our bodies absorb and simulate minerals. What's the benefit of taking a multivitamin every day if your body sees it as a foreign toxin and immediately starts trying to remove it? The answer is hindering the outcome more than helping it (not to mention the complete waste of money).

The most powerful supplement and by far the best multivitamin is always natural food. Hippocrates said it best: "Let thy food be thy medicine and thy medicine be thy food."

If and when you choose a multivitamin (or any vitamin or mineral, for that matter), try to make sure it's raw and sourced from whole plant ingredients. That type of multivitamin can be absorbed by your body much more easily because the ingredients are naturally sourced.

Garden of Life is one of the best companies for naturally sourced supplements that are easy to take and made up of 100 percent plant-based ingredients. Please see `www.gardenoflife.com` for more information.

Supplements may have side effects, including diarrhea or other detoxification symptoms, so be sure to look into these before taking anything.

Consulting with your doctor versus self-prescribing

People love to prescribe themselves supplements. Walking into a health-food store, ordering online, or taking a friend's referral of the "best" things to take may all sound appealing and exciting. But buyer beware! Natural supplements can cause health risks, too. Just because you can buy them over the counter doesn't mean they can be taken by anyone at any time. Some are extremely potent and can aggravate certain conditions or contraindicate other medications or things going on in your body. Many products and supplements sold under the label of "natural" can interact with medications or make certain conditions worse if used inappropriately.

Luckily, health practitioners such as integrative doctors, naturopaths, and clinical nutritionists have studied long and hard about supplements and how and when to take them.

You may find many reasons to consider seeing a naturopathic doctor about supplementation, whether you're dealing with a current illness, concerned about preventing future disease, or simply interested in pursuing a higher level of health. Naturopathic doctors are trained to understand these therapies and the risks involved in them, and they also understand the pathology underlying symptoms to guide appropriate treatment. Naturopaths treat the individual, not the disease. Symptoms viewed in isolation can appear to be identical in different people, but the cause of those symptoms may be completely different.

Naturopathic medicine works best for people who want to have control over how they feel. These health-care practitioners guide you toward better choices, but the choice always remains in your hands.

Choosing plant-based over synthetic supplements

The best supplements on the planet are always plant-based and natural. Don't get fooled into thinking synthetic vitamins are the way to go; they waste your money and time and ultimately hurt your health. Although it seems as though countless gimmicks promise the best supplements and the fastest weight loss, really only one method is tried and true: a completely natural approach. When you use natural nutrition or plant-based supplements, your body works best by absorbing and utilizing all the nutrients.

Synthetic vitamins can actually put a burden on your body and immune system instead of helping better your health. This is because your body sees synthetic vitamins as toxins or threats and starts eliminating them instead of using them — hence the stomachaches or discolored urine you may have when taking them. These supplements are often found at drugstores and club-based warehouse stores. The supplements you want can typically be found at small health- or natural-food stores (or sometimes even online).

Avoid supplements that use words ending in -acid, -ide, and sometimes -ate, or that have the letters "DL" before their name. These indicate that the supplement is synthetic.

Supplements of good quality aren't cheap, but because you're spending the money, why not choose the very best for you and your family that you possibly can and see the greatest results in the long run? You want to seek out nutrition that your body sees as being food and that doesn't set off your white blood cells in defense mode. All in all, supplements are more popular and more complicated than ever, so it's important to remember what really makes them work: high-quality, 100 percent natural plant-based ingredients (without any filler ingredients) that your body recognizes as either food sources or nutrients. This gives you a great absorption rate and maximum utilization in the body.

Watch out for these toxic filler ingredients in your supplements: hydrogenated oils, artificial colors, magnesium stearate, and titanium dioxide.

Don't be penny wise and pound foolish. Scrimping on cost and quality defeats the purpose of taking vitamins and supplements.

Thinking about absorption

The absorption rate of nutrients from your diet and supplements is extremely important when it comes to reaping their health benefits. The quality of your health isn't dependent only on what you eat or ingest but also on *how well your body breaks things down* to get what is needed for optimal health.

Absorption may not seem like an important concept if you're not used to using vitamins or supplements, but it's critical when it comes to truly getting everything out of the nutrition your body needs to be healthy. Absorption is much easier and much more complete at the cellular level when the food or supplement is plant-based because all the enzymes and amino acids are present in their full and natural sequence, and your body can fully absorb all plant-based nutritional supplements without leaving anything to waste. That in turn creates a situation where your body is using these nutrients for their intended purposes.

Focusing on the Main Plant-Based Supplements

When transitioning to a plant-based diet, you need to make sure you get plenty of certain nutrients and vitamins. You can acquire most of them through your new diet of whole foods, but sometimes you may need to take supplements. These additions act as insurance that the body is getting what it needs to function at its best.

This doesn't necessarily mean that you should be on these supplements indefinitely, but definitely for a period of time while your body adjusts to your new lifestyle and builds up its stores. Read on to find out more. If you feel like you're coming up short in consuming any of the nutrient-rich foods I mention, you probably want to talk to your health-care provider.

Please note that these are just guidelines and suggestions about which supplements may be beneficial on a plant-based diet. Please talk to your health practitioner *before* beginning any supplemental protocol.

B vitamins

The family of B vitamins is a big one for plant-based eaters. You need to make sure you're getting enough of them in your diet (luckily they're plentiful in the plant-based food world); otherwise, you may need some additional supplementation.

Of all the B vitamins, vitamin B12 (methylcobalamin) is likely the only one you need to supplement *regularly* as a plant-based eater. It helps in the formulation of normal red blood cells, increases energy, and alleviates psychological symptoms in older people. Food sources that provide B12 include fermented soy products (miso and tempeh) and some sprouts.

Food sources of B12 alone don't provide enough of the vitamin for plant-based eaters, which is why a supplemental form may be necessary.

If you have compromised kidneys, avoid the most commonly available form of B12, cyanocobalamin. Cyanocobalamin contains a small amount of cyanide. People with chronic kidney failure don't detoxify cyanide as well as people with healthy kidneys do, so they should avoid this form. If your kidneys are healthy, you don't have to worry; the amount of cyanide attached to the cobalamin is too small to do any harm.

If you aren't eating enough foods that are rich in B vitamins (see Chapter 3 for more about the B family of vitamins and their food sources), make sure to talk to your health-care provider about possible supplementation with a B-complex vitamin.

Vitamin D

Vitamin D (calciferol) is known as the sunshine vitamin, because it's manufactured from a form of cholesterol in human skin when it comes into contact with UVB light. Vitamin D is rather difficult to get from a plant-based diet, and therefore you may need to take it in supplemental form from time to time.

Vitamin D in general is beneficial for these reasons:

- Helps regulate calcium and phosphorus metabolism and normal calcification of the bones and teeth
- Helps increase the absorption of calcium from the intestines
- Decreases excretion of calcium from the intestines
- Stimulates reabsorption of calcium and phosphorus from bones
- Helps put calcium and phosphorus into the teeth

Vitamin D may also prevent cancer, heart disease, and diabetes.

The most natural and best form of vitamin D comes from the sun; ideally, you'd get at least 20 minutes of sunshine a day between the hours of 10 a.m. and 2 p.m. when the UV index is 3 or higher. How much vitamin D your body produces from sun exposure varies depending on your skin color and where you live (people in Mexico can get more sun exposure more often than people in Canada).

Supplemental vitamin D comes in two forms:

- ✔ **Ergocalciferol (vitamin D$_2$):** Plant-based and derived from yeast. Although vitamin D$_2$ is plant-based and is often prescribed by doctors, this form of vitamin D isn't naturally produced in the body. Therefore, it's not as effective.

- ✔ **Cholecalciferol (vitamin D$_3$):** Animal-based and derived from sheep's wool. The body produces this form of vitamin D naturally through sunshine. Because this form isn't plant-based, take the supplement form only if needed or recommended by your health-care practitioner.

If your health-care practitioner recommends that you take a vitamin D$_3$ supplement, you should take approximately 400 international units (IUs) per day.

If you're taking vitamin D orally, note that it's a fat-soluble vitamin, which means it's stored in the body's fat tissue. Therefore, it's best to take your vitamin D supplement with some sort of dietary fat, such as nuts, seeds, avocados, or healthy oils (such as olive oil), so it can be absorbed into your system. Other fat-soluble vitamins include vitamins A, E, and K.

Step away from the calcium supplements!

Calcium supplements seem to be one of the most popular supplements, whether prescribed by a health-care provider or self-prescribed. The problem is that the calcium in many supplements causes more damage than good. Instead of facilitating calcium storage as intended, these synthetic forms of calcium actually cause mineral loss from bones. They can also lead to a buildup of calcium deposits in the body, which are the leading cause of most major diseases.

So this is one supplement I absolutely *do not* recommend taking in pill, powder, or other processed forms (such as candies and chews).

The only way to absorb the purest form of calcium is through plant-based whole foods. See Chapter 3 for more on which foods are best. It's also important to get regular and adequate sun exposure to maintain optimum vitamin D levels, thereby increasing calcium absorption.

What your body actually needs is magnesium to absorb all the calcium circulating in the body. Luckily, the plant world is full of diverse sources of magnesium, from dark leafy greens to nuts and beans. However, it may be good for aging women to take an extra dose (in liquid supplement form) for bone health.

Choosing the Best Form for Your Supplements

Supplements come in many forms, the main ones being powders, pills, and nutrition bars. You can choose the form based on personal preference, but you should be aware of the pros and cons of each. Read on to get to know some of them better before you take them.

Powders

Powders (which ultimately turn into liquid supplements) are the least convenient to use because they must be mixed into a liquid, shake, or other food. On the other hand, powders do offer great flexibility with dosing — you can make much finer adjustments to the dose than with tablets and capsules — and they're generally easy for people to swallow. Also, many powders contain the same nutrients taken from whole-food sources. Some varieties provide a concentrated amount of nutrients in a small dose that is sometimes more potent than the food source. At the same time, other powders are more refined and will never compare to eating the whole food.

Some people favor liquid supplements based on the belief that liquid supplements absorb more quickly and are therefore better than other forms. They may, but this difference may not be great enough to amount to a noticeable or significant nutritional difference.

Drawbacks? They're always more expensive on a dollars-per-nutrient basis, and their shelf life is shorter than other forms'. Also, many powders have trace amounts of dairy, such as milk powder or whey, so they don't always work for someone trying to stick to plant-based guidelines. Be sure to look closely at any added or non-active ingredients on the label.

Pills

Pills are the most cost-effective supplements in general because they're less expensive to manufacture than other formats, and that cost savings is passed on to you. You can compare two kinds of pills:

- **Tablets** are either chewable or dissolvable and are typically made from powder compacted into a pill form.
- **Capsules** are filled with a liquid or powder and have a smoother coating, making them easier to swallow.

Pills are the most common form of supplements at most health-food stores. They're also easy to pack when you travel as long as you take only the amount you need for the trip and not the whole bottle. Lastly, they're low maintenance and have a pretty good shelf life. Just be sure to check their expiration dates when you purchase them.

Vegetarian capsules, of which Vegicaps are the best-known brand, are a gelatin-free alternative rapidly gaining popularity as customers become more hesitant to consume animal byproducts like gelatin. Some people like the fact that they can open up the capsules and mix the contents into applesauce or a protein shake, for example, instead of swallowing the capsule.

Drawbacks? Many pills are synthetically derived and are made with fillers (that don't do much for your body), and your body only absorbs a small amount of what's in them. So people end up popping more pills than they need (usually the cheaper ones) and at the same time putting unnatural fillers in their bodies — sometimes even animal-derived byproducts, such as milk powders and gelatin.

Bars

Nutrition bars, nut bars, and protein bars, oh my! You can find many supplement bars on the market, many of which you can use as a simple, on-the-go meal replacement or snack when you're in a pinch. However, many of them are highly processed with ingredients you don't want to even think about putting in your body.

Many bars are made from naturally derived whole-food ingredients. Of course, you need to be a good label reader and make sure that you recognize everything in the bar. I favor bars that are made from raw whole foods like nuts, seeds, dried fruit, greens powders, and other healthy, recognizable plant-based ingredients.

Different bars have different ratios of protein, carbohydrates, and fat. Depending on what you're looking for, you should choose your bar accordingly. Is your bar replacing a snack or dinner, or are you looking for a way to get more vitamins in your system? Just be sure that the protein is coming from plant-based sources, such as brown rice, hemp, rice protein, or nuts and seeds.

You have to watch out even for some plant-based protein bars. Many contain added sugars and artificial ingredients and are expensive. Also, many low-carbohydrate protein bars have artificial sweeteners to reduce the calorie content. Furthermore, some protein bars contain fractionated palm-kernel oil, which is naturally high in saturated fats. Fractionating the oil further increases the saturated-fat content by heating and cooling the oil to remove the unsaturated fatty acids. The last and most common ingredient to avoid in a supplement bar is soy protein isolate. This is a highly processed ingredient to avoid even though it is plant-based. It can be carcinogenic and interferes with calcium balance.

Whole-food nutrition always comes first. Only use a bar as a meal replacement in situations that call for it, such as being stuck in traffic or caught in a late meeting, or as a healthy snack alternative to the vending machine. You can get too much of some vitamins and minerals and miss out on the health benefits of whole foods if you consume multiple bars per day. Make sure your protein-bar consumption doesn't replace a balanced diet of fruits, vegetables, and healthy fats.

Picking the Right Times to Supplement

Supplements are supplements for a reason and are meant to be taken in certain situations and at certain times for optimal efficiency and absorption. Then, of course, lifestyle factors sometimes come into play and affect when and what you need. This section outlines when you should take different supplements.

These are just suggestions of the best times to take supplements if you're on a supplement protocol laid out by your health practitioner. If you don't need to take any supplements, you shouldn't.

The one thing to take daily: Probiotics

Probiotics are consumable bacteria that have significant health benefits. Our gut requires a certain amount of healthy bacteria to thrive. So much of this bacteria is lost through a poor diet, the environment, prescriptions, and other external sources that we need to constantly resupply our gut. There's no harm in taking one to two pills of probiotics daily in addition to eating a diet that is high in raw and fermented fruits and vegetables, which contain both *probiotics* (healthy gut flora) and *prebiotics* (healthy gut flora food). With regular intake from whole foods and good supplements, you may experience benefits such as regular bowel movements, less bloating, and better breakdown of food passing through.

You've likely heard a lot about probiotics, typically as acidophilus in commercial dairy yogurt. Well, obviously that doesn't work for you as a plant-based eater. Some nondairy yogurts are made from coconut milk or other alternative milks that contain acidophilus cultures, but unless you make them at home (see *Fermenting For Dummies*), it's likely never the same amount that you can get from a supplement.

Not only that, but the count of bacteria in food doesn't quite compare to what can be found in a supplement. In fact, often a probiotic starter is used to start a culture of yogurt and other fermented foods. You can typically pick these supplements up at any health-food store in the refrigerated section, depending on the brand. Just make sure that it's 100 percent plant-based (watch out for dairy).

As you may know, you can get an extra dose of probiotics from fermented foods, such as unpasteurized sauerkraut, fresh miso paste, and homemade kombucha. Probiotics are naturally occurring in fermented foods and can give your body an extra boost in addition to the supplemental form.

When it's morning

The best time of day to take a multivitamin — if you happen to be taking a high-quality, plant-based version — is usually in the morning, with your first meal. Taking it in the morning allows for the best chance that it'll be absorbed into your system with the food you eat throughout the day.

Another type of vitamin you want to take in the morning is water-soluble vitamins, such as vitamins C and B, which aren't stored in the body's fat tissue and — only if needed — must be replaced each day.

B vitamins are known as the "energy vitamins," so it's definitely better to take them in the morning, because taking them at night can interfere with a good night's sleep.

When you're battling a cold

Everyone wants to know how to prepare for battle when he feels that first sign of a cold coming on, so here are some basic suggestions for things you may want to consider taking when you get that tickle in your throat:

- **Oil of oregano:** It comes in liquid/tincture form. It can be dropped under the tongue or dissolved in water.
- **Vitamin C:** You can take it in capsule, tablet, or liquid form.
- **Zinc:** You can take it in liquid or tablet form.

For specific dosages, follow the indications on the product packaging.

When you have a nutritional deficiency

Seeing your doctor or naturopath can help you better determine which vitamins you need to supplement with. Getting blood work done can best indicate which vital vitamins and minerals your body is missing. That way, you can supplement correctly for your deficiency.

If you have a severe health condition, don't self-medicate. Your doctor or naturopath should give you individual instructions about when you should be taking your supplements and whether to take them with or without a certain kind of food. That way, the supplements best help your deficiency.

When you're on vacation

It's always a wise move to bring your daily supplements on vacation. When you're on vacation, you don't always eat the most nutritious foods. Therefore, bringing your supplements can help your energy, mood, and overall health while you're away from home. Sometimes you want to take specific supplements to certain destinations, and often a health practitioner can advise you on this.

Some of the best supplements to travel with (for emergencies) are:

- ✔ Oil of oregano
- ✔ Probiotics
- ✔ Vitamin C
- ✔ B-complex vitamins
- ✔ A plant-based multivitamin

Part III
Plant-Based Recipes for Success

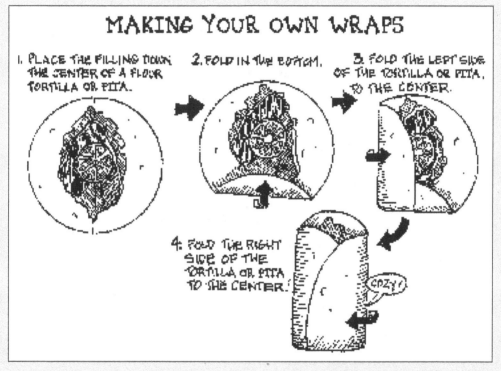

Illustration by Elizabeth Kurtzman

Think you have no time for breakfast? Think again. If you have five minutes, you can whip up a delicious and healthy smoothie. Find out how in the free article at www.dummies.com/extras/plantbaseddiet.

In this part . . .

- ✔ Start your day with plant-based alternatives to eggs and bacon.

- ✔ Check out salad, soup, and nori roll recipes that give you a midday plant-based boost.

- ✔ Create incredible stir-fries, pasta dishes, and other entrees to nourish yourself at the end of the day.

- ✔ Satisfy your sweet tooth with healthy plant-based desserts that derive their sweetness from natural forms of sugar.

- ✔ Try your hand at making sensational snacks.

- ✔ Enhance your meals with delicious plant-based sauces, sides, dressings, and dips.

Chapter 10

Brilliant Breakfasts

*Y*ou've heard it before, and you know it's true: The key to a successful, highly energized day is eating a balanced breakfast. When you get the right plant-based foods into your body in the morning, you feel great — both mentally and physically. Knowing you have great options and feeling fantastic make you ready to tackle the day like a champion.

This chapter outlines several recipes for the most important meal of the day. Start off right with these morning delights and see where the day takes you.

Wakey, Wakey, No Eggs and Bakey

You won't find any egg, sausage, or bacon recipes, or any other animal-based options, in this book. "So then what do I eat for breakfast?" you may be asking. Just wait — this chapter is packed with powerful plant-based breakfast selections that fuel you up, give you energy, and don't weigh you down.

The standard, traditional breakfast of bacon and eggs — although it may be familiar and taste great — is heavy and high in salt and saturated fat. It can leave you feeling uncomfortable and doesn't provide the energy and vigor you need to thrive all day long. However, the good news is that there are many plant-based substitutes for your favorite breakfast items.

⮞ **Eggs:** Opt for a plant-based protein, such as sprouted tofu.

⮞ **Sausage and bacon:** Choose marinated tempeh or baked tofu.

⮞ **Yogurt:** Go with coconut yogurt, chia cereal, or mashed bananas.

⮞ **Milk:** Try almond milk, hempseed milk, rice milk, or coconut milk.

Whether you have a sweet or savory tooth in the morning, it's just a matter of finding the right foods to give you your fix for the day. If you don't get balanced ingredients in your body first thing in the morning, you can set yourself up for cravings, bloating, and general ickiness.

Easy to Make and Easy on the Go

If you want one meal to be easy and quick during the workweek, it's breakfast. Often, this meal gets neglected because of limited time or poor planning. I often hear people complain that they don't eat a good breakfast because they don't have time or they think that making a decent breakfast is too complicated.

You can do a number of things to simplify breakfast preparation and make sure you start your day strongly:

- ✔ Make some or all of your breakfast the night before, such as a smoothie, soaked chia seeds, or oatmeal.

- ✔ Always have nut or seed milk ready to go in the fridge to use as a base for smoothies and porridges — or to add to tea or coffee.

- ✔ Make a batch of muffins whenever you have time (perhaps during the weekend) and store them in the freezer. Then you can pull them out as needed for a simple breakfast.

- ✔ If you like multiple-ingredient breakfasts, measure and portion out ingredients the night before. Store them in their own containers in the fridge or cupboard so they can be easily dumped into a bowl of oatmeal or a blender when you're half asleep.

- ✔ Use glass or stainless-steel storage containers or glass water bottles for taking items on the go. These containers don't leak and keep your breakfast fresh.

- ✔ Save the more involved recipes, such as tofu scrambles and pancakes, for the weekend when you have more time. Or, make extra so you can warm up the leftovers the next day for a simple breakfast.

Try these super-simple ideas for a breakfast with no recipe required:

- ✔ Two slices of whole-grain or sprouted-grain bread with nut or seed butter

- ✔ A banana with a handful of nuts

- ✔ Coconut yogurt topped with fruit

- ✔ Apple slices with almond butter

- ✔ Avocado spread on toast

Homemade Hempseed Milk

Prep time: 5 min • **Yield:** 6 servings

Ingredients	Directions
1 cup hempseeds	*1* Place all the ingredients in a high-speed blender and blend for at least 1 minute.
4 cups water	
1 tablespoon coconut oil	
2 tablespoons maple syrup or coconut nectar	
1 teaspoon vanilla-bean powder, or ½ teaspoon vanilla extract	
1 teaspoon cinnamon	

Per serving: Calories 263 (From Fat 189); Fat 21g (Saturated 26g); Cholesterol 0mg; Sodium 6mg; Carbohydrate 9g (Dietary Fiber 4 g); Protein 13g.

Vary It! Try swapping out the hempseeds for almonds, Brazil nuts, sunflower seeds, or macadamia nuts. If you swap out the hempseeds for a nut with skins, you'll need to strain the milk with a fine mesh colander, cheese cloth, or nut-milk bag to remove the skins from the liquid.

Note: This milk can be stored for up to four days and keeps best in the refrigerator in a glass jar.

Tip: You can substitute this milk measure for measure in most recipes that call for dairy milk.

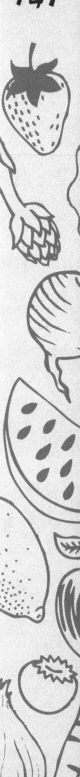

Liquid Nutrition Smoothie

Prep time: 4 min • **Yield:** 2 servings

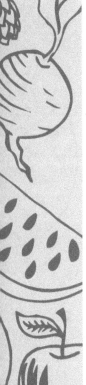

Ingredients	Directions
2 cups rice milk, almond milk, or hempseed milk	*1* Blend all the ingredients in a blender until the mixture is smooth and no lumps remain.
2 to 4 tablespoons plant-based protein powder (such as Sunwarrior or Vega)	*2* Pour into two glasses and enjoy.
½ cup blueberries or mixed berries, fresh or frozen	
1 banana	
½ cup chopped mango, peach, or pear, fresh or frozen	
½ cup ice	
1 teaspoon coconut nectar or raw honey	
½ to 1 cup packed fresh spinach leaves	

Per serving: Calories 186 (From Fat 27); Fat 3g (Saturated 0g); Cholesterol 0mg; Sodium 283mg; Carbohydrate 31g (Dietary Fiber 4g); Protein 11g.

Note: The smoothie will keep for eight hours in the refrigerator.

Vary It! Try adding a tablespoon of any of these superfoods: goji berries, cacao nibs, coconut oil, flax oil, chia seeds, hempseeds, carob powder, maca, matcha green-tea powder, almond butter, or acai-berry powder.

Tip: This smoothie will be creamier if your fruit is frozen, so opt for frozen fruit whenever possible (or just add more ice).

Blueberry Buckwheat Pancakes

Prep time: 10 min • **Cook time:** 25 min • **Yield:** 4–6 servings

Ingredients	Directions
2 cups sifted buckwheat flour	*1* In a small bowl, combine the buckwheat flour, baking powder, salt, baking soda, and maple crystals. Set aside.
½ teaspoon baking powder	
½ teaspoon salt	
1 teaspoon baking soda	*2* In a large bowl, combine the apple-cider vinegar and rice milk. Let sit for 5 to 10 minutes, then add the mashed banana.
2 teaspoons maple crystals or coconut sugar	
3 tablespoons apple-cider vinegar	*3* Add the dry ingredients to the wet ingredients. Beat only until blended.
2 cups rice milk	*4* Add the blueberries.
1 to 2 very ripe bananas, mashed	*5* Heat the coconut oil on a griddle. Using a 1-ounce ladle, pour the batter onto the greased griddle. Cook the pancakes until the bubbles in the batter break on the surface; flip and cook until browned. Repeat until you're out of batter.
1 cup fresh or frozen organic blueberries	
1 tablespoon coconut oil	
	6 Serve on a plate and top with maple syrup, cinnamon, fresh fruit, coconut yogurt, or cashew cream.

Per serving: Calories 349 (From Fat 63); Fat 7g (Saturated 3g); Cholesterol 0mg; Sodium 701mg; Carbohydrate 65g (Dietary Fiber 10g); Protein 12g.

Vary It! Try these pancakes with different fruits, such as cranberries or strawberries, or make them even more decadent by adding some non-dairy chocolate chips. You can also substitute another gluten-free or whole-grain flour such as brown rice or oat flour for the buckwheat flour.

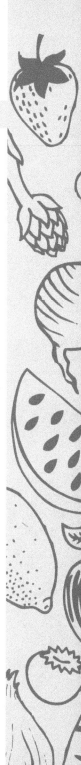

Apple Cinnamon Mini-Muffins

Prep time: 15 min • **Cook time:** 12 min • **Yield:** 12–20 mini-muffins

Ingredients	Directions
1 cup spelt flour, kamut flour, or oat flour	**1** Preheat the oven to 350 degrees.
½ cup rolled oats	**2** Combine the dry ingredients in a large bowl. Set aside.
1 teaspoon baking powder	
½ teaspoon baking soda	**3** Combine the wet ingredients and apples in a medium bowl.
¼ teaspoon cinnamon	
¼ teaspoon sea salt	**4** Pour the wet ingredients into the dry ingredients and mix well, making sure there are no lumps. Stir in the raisins.
¼ cup coconut oil or grape-seed oil	
¼ cup maple syrup	**5** Distribute the mixture evenly in a 24-cup mini-muffin pan. You can use coconut oil or grapeseed oil to grease the tin, or use paper liner cups.
⅓ cup applesauce	
½ cup rice milk	
1 apple, seeded and cut into small cubes	**6** Bake for 12 minutes.
½ cup raisins	**7** Remove the pan from the oven and let it sit for a few minutes, then remove the muffins and cool them on a cooling rack or tray.

Per serving: Calories 140 (From Fat 45); Fat 5g (Saturated 4g); Cholesterol 0mg; Sodium 115mg; Carbohydrate 22g (Dietary Fiber 2g); Protein 2g.

Note: Be sure to use unbleached parchment-paper cups. These are brown, not white. You don't want any residue leaching into your tasty muffins!

Vary It! Use this recipe to make 8 to 12 full-sized muffins — just be sure to extend the baking time to 20 minutes. You can also swap in a gluten-free flour, such as brown-rice flour.

Tip: If you have empty muffin cups after filling the cups with batter, add water to the empty cups to prevent burning.

Morning Millet Granola

Prep time: 8 min • **Cook time:** 25 min • **Yield:** Approx 6 cups

Ingredients	Directions
¾ cup pure organic maple syrup	**1** Preheat the oven to 300 degrees.
1 tablespoon rice milk	**2** Combine the maple syrup, rice milk, and coconut oil in a large saucepan and set aside.
¼ cup coconut oil	
4 cups rolled oats	**3** Mix the remaining ingredients, except the raisins, in a large bowl. Toss well.
1½ cups puffed millet cereal or millet flakes	
¾ cup sesame seeds	**4** Add the syrup mixture and stir well.
½ cup sunflower seeds	**5** Pour the mixture into two shallow pans or baking sheets lined with parchment paper and bake for 15 minutes. Stir, then bake for an additional 10 minutes.
½ cup pumpkin seeds	
1 cup unsweetened coconut flakes	
¼ cup flaxseeds	**6** Take the granola out of the oven and add the raisins.
1 cup chopped almonds	
1 teaspoon sea salt	**7** Cool and store in an airtight container.
1½ cups raisins, apricots, or cranberries (unsulphured)	

Per serving: Calories 281 (From Fat 117); Fat 13g (Saturated 4.5g); Cholesterol 0mg; Sodium 73mg; Carbohydrate 41g (Dietary Fiber 5g); Protein 5g.

Note: Don't add the raisins or other dried fruits too early — they get very hard if baked in the oven.

Vary It! Instead of millet, you can use oat bran, quinoa, or amaranth flakes.

Tip: Serve this granola with coconut yogurt and top it with fresh berries for a hearty breakfast delight.

Note: Be sure that the dried fruit you buy is sulphite free. Suphates are preservatives that keep fruit "fresh" long after it has been harvested. Always check to make sure the dried fruit you buy is free of this additive.

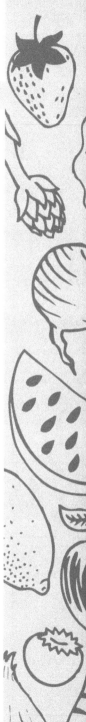

Soaked Oats with Goji Berries

Prep time: 10 min plus soaking time • **Cook time:** 2–10 min • **Yield:** 1–2 servings

Ingredients	Directions
½ cup whole rolled oats	*1* Combine the oats, water, and lemon juice in a bowl. Cover with a plate and soak overnight at room temperature.
½ cup water	
1 tablespoon fresh-squeezed lemon juice	*2* For cold oats, add the remaining ingredients to the bowl and enjoy.
½ cup rice milk or almond milk	
1 tablespoon almond butter	*3* For warm oats, add all the ingredients to a pot with an additional splash of rice milk. Warm for 5 minutes and serve.
1 banana, sliced	
2 tablespoons goji berries	
1 teaspoon cinnamon	
¼ cup pumpkin seeds	
1 tablespoon maple syrup	

Per serving: Calories 433 (From Fat 144); Fat 16g (Saturated 2.5g); Cholesterol 0mg; Sodium 49mg; Carbohydrate 62g (Dietary Fiber 6g); Protein 15g.

Note: If you like your raisins or pumpkin seeds soft, soak them overnight with the oats. If you want to make the warming process even easier, prepare this recipe in a slow cooker the night before and just turn the heat on in the morning for a few minutes to warm it up.

Vary It! Try using some of these toppings instead for a different flavor: chia seeds, sunflower seeds, walnuts, currents, apple slices, pear slices, cacao nibs, or hempseeds.

Super Chia Banana Porridge

Prep time: 10 min • **Cook time:** 15 min • **Yield:** 1 serving

Ingredients	Directions
¼ **cup chia seeds, soaked in** ½ **cup water or hempseed milk for 10 minutes**	*1* Stir the soaked chia seeds until a gel-like consistency forms. Add a bit more liquid if desired.
½ **to 1 ripe banana, mashed**	*2* Add the mashed banana. Combine until the mixture has a porridge-like consistency.
1 teaspoon cinnamon	
1 teaspoon green powder (optional)	*3* Stir in the cinnamon, green powder (if desired), coconut oil or nut butter, and berries.
1 tablespoon softened coconut oil or nut butter	
2 tablespoons fresh berries	*4* Serve in a bowl and enjoy. Top with coconut flakes for extra crunch.

Per serving: *Calories 382 (From Fat 243); Fat 27g (Saturated 13g); Cholesterol 0mg; Sodium 11mg; Carbohydrate 33g (Dietary Fiber 16g); Protein 8g.*

Tip: The ideal amount of time to soak chia is approximately 10 minutes for a thick consistency; for an even thicker consistency, soak it longer. If you want it thinner, add more liquid.

Note: Green powders come in many varieties. Aim for a single-source powder such as chlorella, spirulina, or hemp powder, or blends that contain only green ingredients. This ensures that you aren't getting any other additives.

Vary It! Try sunflower-seed butter or cashew butter instead of coconut oil for a variation. Also try adding a scoop of protein powder or topping the mixture with hempseeds, goji berries, or pumpkin seeds for an extra boost of protein.

Tip: This breakfast is great on the go — you can get it ready the night before and have it ready to take with you in the morning.

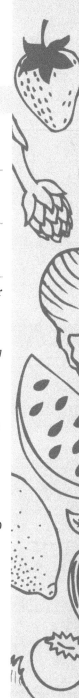

Amaranth Porridge with Fruit Compote

Prep time: 25 min, plus soaking time • **Cook time:** 20–30 min • **Yield:** 4 servings

Ingredients	Directions
Fruit Compote (see the following recipe) 1 cup dried amaranth 2 tablespoons fresh-squeezed lemon juice 3 cups water ½ teaspoon sea salt 1 tablespoon freshly ground flax, or other nuts or seeds	**1** Place enough water in a bowl to cover the amaranth. Add the lemon juice and soak the grain overnight. Rinse and drain the amaranth in the morning and place into a pot with 3 cups of fresh water.
	2 Bring it to a boil, add the sea salt, reduce the heat to low, cover, and simmer for 20 to 30 minutes. Remove from the heat.
	3 Dish into bowls, sprinkle flax or nuts on top, and top with the Fruit Compote.

Fruit Compote

2 firm pears

1 teaspoon fresh-squeezed lemon juice in 3 cups of water

½ cup dried apricots

4 dried figs

½ cup raisins or dried cranberries

2 cups apple juice

½ cup rice syrup

2 large pieces of lemon peel

1 teaspoon coconut oil

pinch of sea salt

In a tea bag:

1 cinnamon stick

3 whole cloves

1 teaspoon ground anise

1-inch piece of ginger

1 Peel, core, and slice the pears into ¼-inch pieces. Place them in the lemon water and set aside. Slice the apricots and figs into ½-inch slices.

2 In a medium saucepan, bring the apple juice, rice syrup, lemon peel, coconut oil, and sea salt to a boil. Lower the heat and simmer about 3 minutes.

3 Add the tea bag to the simmering liquid. Gently stir in the pears (discarding the liquid in which they were soaking), apricots, figs, and cranberries and continue to simmer uncovered on medium heat for about 15 minutes.

4 Remove the tea bag. Strain the liquid into a small saucepan and set the fruit mixture aside in a bowl.

5 Boil the liquid until it's syrupy and reduced to about 1 cup. Remove from the heat. Serve chilled or warm.

Per serving: Calories 512 (From Fat 54); Fat 6g (Saturated 1.5g); Cholesterol 0mg; Sodium 726mg; Carbohydrate 113g (Dietary Fiber 10g); Protein 9g.

Vary It! Instead of the compote, try serving the porridge with almond milk, rice milk, coconut milk, maple syrup, coconut nectar, or raw honey.

Tip: You can buy empty tea bags that you can fill yourself at home; be sure to buy ones without any bleach. Alternatively, you can use a tea infuser.

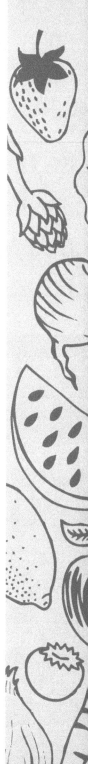

Turmeric Tofu Scramble

Prep time: 5 min • **Cook time:** 20 min • **Yield:** 6 servings

Ingredients	Directions
1 tablespoon ground cumin	*1* In a small bowl, mix together the cumin, turmeric, coriander, chili powder (if desired), paprika, thyme, cayenne, salt, and black pepper.
1 tablespoon ground turmeric	
1 teaspoon coriander	
½ teaspoon chili powder (optional)	*2* In a sauté pan, heat the grapeseed oil over medium heat and add the onion, green bell pepper, if desired, and spices. Cook until the onion is softened, about 5 minutes.
½ teaspoon paprika	
1 teaspoon dried thyme	
pinch cayenne pepper	*3* Crumble the tofu into bite-sized pieces with a fork and add it to the sauté pan, Stir to coat the tofu with the spice mixture. Sauté for 5 minutes over medium to high heat.
¼ teaspoon sea salt	
ground black pepper to taste	
1 tablespoon grapeseed oil	
1 onion, peeled and diced	
1 green bell pepper, diced (optional)	
2 pounds firm organic tofu, drained	

Per serving: Calories 185 (From Fat 90); Fat 10g (Saturated 1g); Cholesterol 0mg; Sodium 153mg; Carbohydrate 6g (Dietary Fiber 2.5g); Protein 15g.

Tip: Serve the scramble with some sprouted-grain toast and steamed greens for a balanced breakfast.

Orange Maple Marinated Tempeh

Prep time: 10 min, plus marinating time • **Cook time:** 25 min • **Yield:** 6 servings

Ingredients	Directions
One 8.5-ounce package organic tempeh	*1* Cut the tempeh lengthwise into 10 strips. If it is frozen, thaw it slightly first.
¼ cup fresh-squeezed orange juice	*2* Mix the remaining ingredients in a small bowl to make the marinade.
2 tablespoons tamari	
3 tablespoons olive oil	*3* Place the tempeh in a casserole dish and pour the marinade over it.
1 tablespoon maple syrup	
2 tablespoons minced white or red onion	*4* Marinate in the refrigerator for as little as 1 hour or up to 6 hours.
1 clove garlic, minced	
	5 Bake covered at 350 degrees for 20 minutes. Remove the cover and bake for 10 more minutes or until the marinade is absorbed.

Per serving: Calories 160 (From Fat 90); Fat 10g (Saturated 1.5g); Cholesterol 0mg; Sodium 340mg; Carbohydrate 10g (Dietary Fiber 4 g); Protein 9g.

Note: You can prepare this ahead of time to allow the tempeh to absorb the flavors, or you can prepare it immediately after putting the marinade on it. Either way, it tastes delicious!

Tip: Use this recipe in place of bacon. Serve it alongside the Turmeric Tofu Scramble (see the recipe earlier in this chapter) or with toast, avocado, and steamed spinach to make a delicious breakfast sandwich.

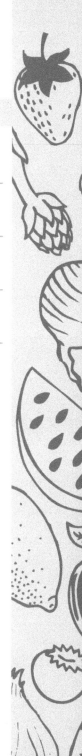

Chapter 11

Lovable Lunches

In This Chapter

▶ Enjoying soups and salads that fill you up

▶ Making meatless sandwiches

▶ Preparing quick lunch dishes

When it comes to lunch, you probably want to just grab something and not spend too much time, if any, prepping it. You can make this easier on yourself — it comes down to proper planning and organization. Lunch recharges you after a busy morning and sets the tone for the rest of the day. You want to make sure it's balanced, varied, and filling enough that it lasts until snack time. (See Chapter 14 for tips about snacks.)

The best way to tackle lunch as a beginning plant-based eater is to make a fantastically filling salad or satisfying soup. Both of these options can be modified with different veggies and enjoyed any time of year; however, you may want to lean more in the salad direction during the warmer months and toward soups in the colder ones.

In this chapter, I give you some great ideas for making simple, quick lunches that you can pack (even in a pinch) and take with you for the workday or out on the town. If you're at home during the day, these are easy go-to meals that you can pull out and put together with very little effort.

Making a Meal of Salads and Soups

Often people think that salads and soups are only precursors to meals, but they can be the centerpieces of your meal. This section tells you how to make intricate and unique salads, along with hearty and filling soups that can eat like a meal!

Making your fridge a salad bar

The best thing you can do to plan proper meals is to get some base ingredients and have them prepped and ready. When hunger strikes, you can just assemble them and go.

What to have ready:

- ✔ **A cooked grain, such as quinoa, rice, or barley.** Be sure to cook your favorite grain ahead of time. Then seal it in a glass container so it's ready to go.

- ✔ **Green leafy veggies, such as arugula, spinach, leaf lettuce, or kale.** These can be washed, stemmed, and chopped and then stored in a perforated bag or glass container.

  Don't leave them too long in the fridge once cut, or they will start to turn brown.

- ✔ **Veggies, like carrots, beets, cucumber, bell peppers, tomatoes, cabbage, and seaweed.** These can all be peeled, chopped, and prepared ahead of time and placed in glass containers for easy use and storage.

- ✔ **Fruit.** Try apples, oranges, avocados, or strawberries. Wash these ahead of time and cut them as you use them.

  If you cut your fruit too early, it is more likely to oxidize and break down. When the flesh is exposed to air, apples and bananas turn brown, berries break down, and other items just get mushy. So the best way to keep your fruit fresh is to cut it right before you use it.

- ✔ **A hearty protein, such as chickpeas, kidney beans, black beans, baked or marinated tofu, or tempeh.** If you're cooking beans from scratch, be sure to rinse them after cooking and store them in a glass container. For tofu and tempeh, you can bake, grill, sauté, or marinate it. Then they're ready to be used on demand.

- ✔ **Herbs and spices.** Parsley, mint, oregano, and basil are always good. Be sure to stock both fresh and dried varieties of different herbs.

- ✔ **Fun toppings, such as hempseeds, pumpkin seeds, sunflower seeds, hazelnuts, cranberries, raisins, or figs.** You can store these in glass jars or small containers and have them ready to go in your pantry.

You can change these items up on a weekly basis, depending on what you have access to, giving yourself a healthy rotation for your own personal salad bar.

Knowing when to use fresh or dried herbs

Many recipes call for herbs. Sometimes they list fresh herbs in the ingredients list, and sometimes they list dried herbs. And sometimes they don't specify which type to use. So when do you use fresh, and when do you used dried?

Fresh herbs are mostly used in dips, salads, and spreads. A recipe may call for them in a cooked dish; if that's the case, the herbs will be added toward the end so as not to destroy all their flavors by cooking.

Dried herbs are best in soups, sauces, and marinades where they have a chance to absorb liquid and transfer their flavor to the dish. Dried herbs are typically added at the beginning or midway through a recipe.

The best way to store any food, cooked or raw, is to seal it in a glass container. Glass is clean, nontoxic, and nonporous, and your food will stay fresher. Plastic containers leach chemicals into your food, they stain easily, and food can spoil more quickly in them. Plastic can also break down over time, whereas glass has a much longer life. Yes, glass may travel a little heavier in your bag, but it is a much healthier and more sustainable choice.

Falling in love with one-pot meals

What could be better than having a full meal, with all of your main nutrients, warmed up in a pot? Soup not only provides your body and brain with a balanced, veggie-happy lunch but also nourishes you for the day.

Here are some general ideas for what to put in a satisfying soup:

- ✔ 4 to 8 cups of liquid base: veggie stock, water, miso paste, herbs, and spices

- ✔ 1 to 3 cups of different veggies, such as carrots, celery, onions, broccoli, onions, kale, spinach, bok choy, zucchini, squash, and Jerusalem artichokes

- ✔ 1 to 2 cups of cooked beans, such as chickpeas, black beans, lentils, white beans, and split peas

- ✔ 1 to 2 cups of cooked whole grains: barley, brown rice, quinoa, or brown-rice pasta

- ✔ ¼ cup of sea vegetables, such as dulse, arame, wakame, or nori

There aren't too many rules with soup, so here are some general steps for getting your soup on:

1. **First warm up the base, usually 4 to 8 cups of liquid.**
2. **Add dense veggies, which typically make up most of the soup.**
3. **Add a protein source, such as a bean or whole grain.**
4. **Add sea vegetables, if desired.** These are usually a small, optional component of a soup unless it's a miso soup (like the Chunky Miso Soup recipe later in this chapter).

Some soups require you to cook your grains and beans before you add them to a soup because they typically don't cook properly in the company of other spices, herbs, and vegetables. It's best to cook them separately in another pot. Then you can add them along the way.

Rethinking Handheld Lunches

Most people love a good, hearty sandwich. When meat is no longer in the picture, people often experience a sense of loss about what can go in between those slices of bread! Well, you have lots of options — more than you can even imagine. But first, a note about bread.

Pick a whole-grain or sprouted-grain bread made from spelt, kamut, oats, or barley. You can even opt for gluten-free breads and wraps made from brown rice, quinoa, or millet flour.

Food for Life, a brand available at most major grocery stores, has amazing sprouted-grain tortillas, brown-rice wraps, and corn tortillas.

When you've chosen your bread, select your stuffings:

- **Protein:** Go with hummus or another bean dip, grilled or baked tofu or tempeh, a veggie burger, falafel, or a Spinach Almond Patty (see Chapter 15 for the recipe).
- **Fat:** Try avocado, cashew cheese, sunflower-seed butter, tahini, or almond butter.
- **Veggies:** Good options include green leafies, sprouts, cucumbers, tomatoes, carrots, beets, onions, mushrooms, or radishes.
- **Dressing:** Try a homemade salad dressing or other marinade, salsa, tomato sauce, Dijon mustard, or avocado spread.

Kale and Cabbage Slaw Salad

Prep time: 5 min • **Cook time:** 30 min • **Yield:** 10–12 servings

Ingredients	Directions
1 head red cabbage	*1* Shred the cabbage, carrots, beet, and fennel in a food processor with a shredding blade, or use a mandolin, or hand slice into thin strips.
2 carrots	
1 beet	
1 head fennel	*2* Remove the stems from the kale, and then chop the kale into thin strips or bite-sized pieces.
1 bunch kale (about 3 cups)	
½ cup olive oil	*3* In a mixing bowl, mix together the olive oil, apple-cider vinegar, lemon juice, and raw honey or coconut nectar to make a vinaigrette.
¼ cup apple-cider vinegar	
Juice of 1 lemon (about 3 to 4 tablespoons)	*4* Combine the vinaigrette with the shredded vegetables and toss until the cabbage and kale are well-coated.
2 tablespoons raw honey or coconut nectar	
2 tablespoons hempseeds	*5* Allow the salad to marinate in the fridge for 30 to 60 minutes.
	6 Mix in the hempseeds just before serving.

Per serving: Calories 178 (From Fat 117); Fat 13g (Saturated 3g); Cholesterol 0mg; Sodium 58mg; Carbohydrate 16g (Dietary Fiber 4g); Protein 4g.

Note: This salad can be consumed right after it's tossed together, but it will taste better and be easier to chew when it marinates longer. It also tastes great the next day!

Vary It! Instead of olive oil, try hemp, pumpkin, or chia oil for variety and a boost of omega-3 fatty acids. You can add sliced avocado on top of this salad to give it a nourishing boost.

Tip: If you are using lacinato kale (dark kale), the stems are much softer and can be chopped into this salad. However, most other varieties such as curly kale or red Russian will need the stems removed.

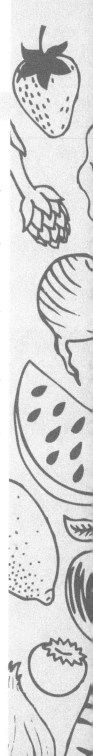

Quinoa Tabbouleh Salad

Prep time: 10 min • **Cook time:** 25 min • **Yield:** 8 servings

Ingredients	Directions
Dressing (see the following recipe)	**1** Rinse the quinoa and strain it through a fine mesh strainer. Add the rinsed quinoa to a pot and heat over medium-low heat for 2 to 3 minutes, or until the moisture has evaporated and it smells kind of nutty. Add water and a pinch of sea salt, bring to a boil, and cover.
1 cup quinoa	
1½ cups water	
Pinch sea salt	
1 cup chickpeas	**2** Lower the heat and simmer the quinoa for 12 to 15 minutes, or until all the water has been absorbed.
½ cup chopped red onion	
¼ cup chopped fresh parsley	**3** Turn off the heat and let the quinoa stand for 2 minutes. Then remove the quinoa and spread it out to cool.
¼ cup chopped fresh mint	
2 cups spinach, finely chopped	**4** Place the quinoa into a bowl and combine with chickpeas, onions, parsley, mint, spinach, cucumber, and tomatoes.
½ cucumber, diced	
1 cup cherry tomatoes, quartered	**5** Add the dressing to the quinoa mixture and gently stir from the bottom up.

Dressing

1 clove of garlic, minced

1 teaspoon dry basil

2 tablespoons lemon juice

1 tablespoon apple-cider vinegar

1 teaspoon honey or coconut nectar

2 teaspoons Dijon mustard

¼ cup olive oil

1 Combine all the ingredients until well mixed.

Per serving: Calories 192 (From Fat 81); Fat 9g (Saturated 1g); Cholesterol 0mg; Sodium 108mg; Carbohydrate 24g (Dietary Fiber 4g); Protein 6g.

Note: Rinse the quinoa well in Step 1 to make it easier to cook and eat. Then dry toast the quinoa to create a better consistency and prevent the quinoa from sticking while it's cooking in Step 2.

Vary It! If tomatoes aren't in season, swap them out for shredded or chopped carrots. Or, try using tahini instead of Dijon mustard in the dressing for a different tabbouleh experience.

Maximizing your leftovers

An easy way to enjoy lunch without doing any extra work during the day is to make more dinner than you need the night before. Then pack up the overflow, and it's ready to go for the next day's lunch. This may require some planning so you can get more ingredients. Items such as pasta, quinoa salads, and noodle dishes keep well in a glass container overnight for lunch the next day.

Another way to maximize your leftovers is having one meal item that can go a long way and be used in different ways. For instance, if you make a bean dip, veggie patty, and guacamole, you can find different ways to enjoy them: in a wrap, on a salad, on top of whole grain, or in pasta. You'll find many ways to use the same ingredient more than once while still getting variety.

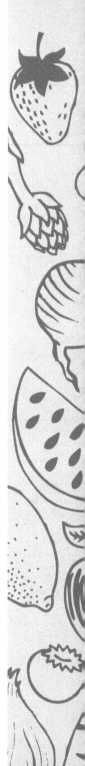

Citrus Wild Rice and Broccoli

Prep time: 10 min • **Cook time:** 45 min • **Yield:** 8 servings

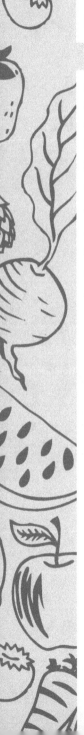

Ingredients	Directions
Vinaigrette (see the following recipe)	*1* Drain the soaked rice and place it in a medium saucepan. Add 2 cups of water and salt and bring to a boil.
1 cup wild rice, soaked overnight in 2 cups of water	
2 cups water	*2* Lower the heat and simmer, covered, until the grains have burst open and are tender but still chewy (about 35 to 45 minutes). Drain and set aside in a medium bowl.
½ teaspoon sea salt	
1 head broccoli	*3* While the rice is cooking, make the vinaigrette.
½ cup sliced or supremed orange segments	*4* Cut the broccoli into small florets and place in a steamer basket over boiling water for 3 minutes or until they're dark green and tender. Run the broccoli under cool water to halt the cooking.
⅓ cup cranberries	
½ cup hazelnuts or pecans	
	5 Pour the vinaigrette over the rice. Add the cranberries, broccoli, orange segments, and nuts to the rice, mix, and serve.

Vinaigrette

2 tablespoons orange zest, or the zest of 1 orange	*1* If you're using fresh zest, zest the orange.
¼ cup fresh-squeezed orange juice	*2* Mix the vinaigrette ingredients together and pour over the warm rice.
2 tablespoons lemon juice	
2 teaspoons balsamic vinegar	
¼ teaspoon ground cinnamon	
½ teaspoon sea salt	
¼ cup olive oil	

Per serving: Calories 200 (From Fat 108); Fat 12g (Saturated 1g); Cholesterol 0mg; Sodium 268mg; Carbohydrate 21g (Dietary Fiber 3g); Protein 5g.

Vary It! Instead of broccoli, try green beans, snap peas, or snow peas for a unique variation.

Note: If you can't get your hands on wild rice, use a long-grain brown rice or wild-rice blend. The salad will taste just as delicious! This salad tastes great both warm and cold out of the fridge.

Also, be sure not to over-steam your broccoli. You want to make sure it's green — not brown — when you place it in your salad.

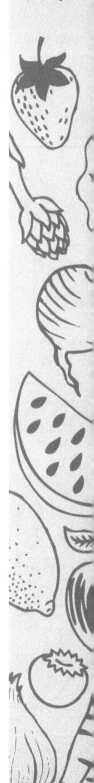

New Age Minestrone

Prep time: 25 min • **Cook time:** 60 min • **Yield:** 12 servings

Ingredients

1 white onion, cut into large cubes

1 clove of garlic, minced

1 tablespoon olive oil

1 teaspoon sea salt

1 tablespoon dried oregano

1 tablespoon dried basil

4 cups water

1 bay leaf

1 butternut squash, peeled and cut into medium cubes

3 parsnips, peeled and cut into medium cubes

1 sweet potato, peeled and cut into large cubes

3 ribs celery, cut into medium pieces

1 large zucchini, cut into small chunks

4 to 5 cups of Swiss chard, cut into bite-sized pieces

1 cup soaked and cooked kidney beans, or one 14-ounce can organic kidney beans

½ cup cooked brown-rice macaroni noodles

Directions

1 In a large pot, sauté the onion and garlic in oil with sea salt until soft.

2 Add the oregano and basil, and sauté for a few more minutes.

3 Add the water and bay leaf.

4 Add the squash, parsnips, and sweet potatoes to the pot. Bring everything to a boil and then reduce the heat to low. Simmer for 10 minutes.

5 Add the celery and zucchini. Turn up the heat again until the water boils and then lower the heat and simmer, covered, for 40 to 45 minutes.

6 Stir the vegetables until the squash falls apart, or press the squash against the side of the pot to break it down.

7 Add the chopped chard. Cover and simmer for 10 minutes.

8 Add the cooked kidney beans and macaroni noodles. Season to taste with salt and pepper. Remove the bay leaf. Stir a few times and serve.

Per serving: *Calories 100 (From Fat 4.5); Fat 1.5g (Saturated 0g); Cholesterol 0mg; Sodium 421mg; Carbohydrate 20g (Dietary Fiber 5g); Protein 4g.*

Tip: Be sure to cook your macaroni noodles al dente in a separate pot so they don't get too hard or too soft. Then add them into the hot soup at the end.

Chunky Miso Soup

Prep time: 10 min • **Cook time:** 40 min • **Yield:** 8–10 servings

Ingredients	Directions

Ingredients

8 cups water

1-inch piece kombu (sea vegetable)

5 dried or fresh shiitake mushrooms

1 small white onion, cut into small slices

2 large carrots, peeled and cut into small pieces

2 to 4 stalks of celery, cut into small pieces

1 block or 12 ounces organic firm tofu, cut into cubes

1 cup chopped bok choy

½ cup wakame (seaweed), soaked for 5 minutes and cut into bite-sized pieces

One 16-ounce package brown rice vermicelli or soba noodles, cooked (optional)

2/3 cup miso paste, brown, white, or both

3 green onions, thinly chopped

Directions

1 Bring 8 cups of water to a boil in a large pot and add the strip of kombu, along with the shiitake mushrooms. (This adds extra nutrients to the soup broth.)

2 Add the onion, carrots, and celery. Reduce the heat to low and let the vegetables simmer for 30 minutes.

3 Add the tofu cubes and simmer for another 10 minutes.

4 Add the bok choy and wakame, allowing it to wilt into the warm soup. Add the cooked noodles (if desired).

5 Remove 1 to 2 cups of the liquid and stir in the miso paste in a separate bowl. When the miso paste is dissolved, pour the mixture back into the soup pot.

6 Ladle the soup into bowls and garnish with fresh green onions.

Per serving: Calories 149 (From Fat 27); Fat 3g (Saturated 0.5g); Cholesterol 0mg; Sodium 919mg; Carbohydrate 23g (Dietary Fiber 3g); Protein 10g.

Note: Always add miso paste at the end. Miso is very delicate and should never be boiled. Boiling destroys all of its natural enzymes.

Tip: There are different varieties of miso. Brown miso is much richer and saltier; white miso is much lighter and sweeter. Try different varieties to see what tastes best to you.

Vary It! All seaweed is loaded with minerals, nutrients, and natural iodine. It is an excellent addition to your soup! If you can't get your hands on wakame, try nori, dulse, or arame.

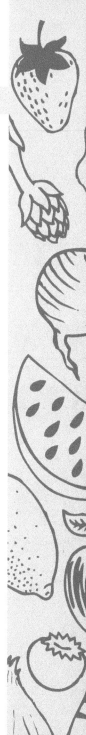

Vegetarian Nori Rolls

Prep time: 30 min • **Cook time:** 30 min • **Yield:** 8 servings

Ingredients	Directions

Ingredients

Vinegar Mixture (see the following recipe)

2 cups short-grain brown rice

4¼ cups water

3 pinches sea salt

3 shiitake mushrooms, stemmed and cut into strips

2 tablespoons maple syrup

3 tablespoons tamari

4 to 6 sheets of raw nori

1 avocado, skinned and sliced

1 small carrot, julienned into long strips

½ cucumber, sliced into thin strips

Wasabi powder, mixed in water to form paste

Pickled ginger

Directions

1 Cook the rice with water and salt for 40 to 50 minutes. Prepare the Vinegar Mixture.

2 Soak the shiitake mushroom strips in maple syrup and tamari for 10 minutes.

3 When the rice is finished cooking, spread it on a cookie sheet with a wooden spoon paddle and cool it by waving a sushi mat back and forth, or place it in the refrigerator.

4 To assemble the rolls, lay a nori sheet flat on the sushi mat with the rough side facing up. Keeping your fingers damp at all times, press rice onto the nori, stopping ¾ inch from the edges. Arrange the vegetables along the bottom of the rice and roll the nori, pressing tight with the mat.

5 Peel the mat away and place the sushi log on a cutting board. Using a sharp knife that's damp, slice the log into 6 to 8 pieces evenly, starting from the center.

6 To serve, place the nori rolls on a plate along with some pickled ginger and wasabi paste.

Vinegar Mixture

2 tablespoons brown-rice
vinegar

2 tablespoons maple syrup

3 tablespoons mirin

½ teaspoon sea salt

1 In a small pot, bring the vinegar, maple syrup, mirin, and salt to a boil; simmer until the salt is dissolved. Cool to room temperature. Sprinkle on cooled rice.

Per serving: Calories 203 (From Fat 18); Fat 2g (Saturated 0g); Cholesterol 0mg; Sodium 634mg; Carbohydrate 47g (Dietary Fiber 4g); Protein 5g.

Note: Soak brown rice overnight for an even creamier texture.

Vary It! Try using different vegetables that are in season, such as green onions, cabbage, radishes, or even fruit such as mango.

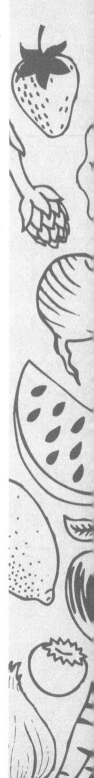

Sun Seed Nori Rolls

Prep time: 20 min • **Cook time:** 15 min • **Yield:** 4–10 servings

Ingredients	Directions
Seed Spread (see the following recipe)	*1* Prepare the Seed Spread.
4 to 6 sheets of raw nori	*2* Lay one nori sheet flat on a surface with the rough side facing up.
1 carrot, shredded	
2 small beets, shredded	*3* Spread about ¼ cup of seed spread on the nori sheet. (You can fill it to the edges if you want.)
½ cucumber, sliced lengthwise	
1 avocado, sliced lengthwise	*4* Place your veggies in a relatively thin horizontal row toward the bottom of the sheet.
Handful of sprouts (mung, sunflower, or pea shoots)	
	5 Roll by lifting the bottom edge closest to you and wrap it over all the veggies. Holding tight, continue to roll it all the way up. Seal it with some water or extra seed spread.
	6 Cut the rolls, using a sharp, damp knife. Start in the center of the roll and keep cutting down the center of each half until you have 6 to 8 pieces.

Seed Spread

1 cup sunflower seeds, soaked for 10 to 12 hours

1 cup almonds, soaked for 10 to 12 hours

1 to 2 tablespoons fresh dill

1 tablespoon fresh oregano

1 teaspoon fresh sage, chopped

2 tablespoons lemon juice

1 tablespoon tamari

1 teaspoon fresh ginger

1 tablespoon dulse granules

½ teaspoon sea salt

1 Place all the spread ingredients in a food processor or high-speed blender and blend until uniform. For a smoother consistency, add a touch of water or blend longer.

Per serving: Calories 494 (From Fat 351); Fat 39g (Saturated 4g); Cholesterol 0mg; Sodium 685mg; Carbohydrate 28g (Dietary Fiber 11g); Protein 18g.

Note: Be sure to use raw nori to make raw nori rolls. (It doesn't work if you buy the toasted kind.)

Tip: This recipe makes a great appetizer at a party and is extremely colorful. Make sure you load your nori rolls up with different veggies each time you make them.

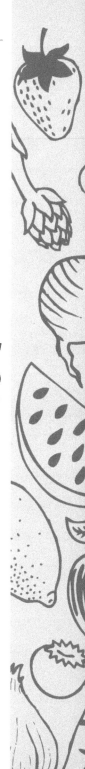

Chapter 12

Super Suppers

In This Chapter

▷ Making wholesome dinners for the whole family

▷ Stretching dinners beyond one meal

▷ Using diversity in recipes to satisfy your appetite

I know — dinner can seem daunting. It's the pinnacle of the day's meals. It's what everyone looks forward to after a hard day of work or school. It's the heartiest and most filling of all meals. But don't panic. Supper in the plant-based world is manageable (and fun!) because you have so many different ways to prepare the same food. It's all about simple creativity!

If you're just starting out on a plant-based diet or simply don't have time to spend all day cooking dinner, consider cooking more food than you need for one meal and then building your next dinner around the leftovers. The good news is that most plant-based foods last longer in the fridge than meat because they don't have the same bacteria issues. Better yet, some items can even be frozen. That way, on busy weeknights, you can just pull out a soup or stew from the freezer, make a fresh salad or steam greens or grains as an easy side component, and voilá — a full, super supper is served!

Don't leave items in the freezer too long; they'll not only lose their nutrients but also get freezer burn and have to be thrown out. On average, consider a freezer time of no more than three months.

Rethinking What Your Dinner Plate Should Look Like

When it comes to dinnertime — whether you're cooking for one, three, or five — it's important to think about versatility and variety. Make sure everyone in the family is satisfied. A typical plate that many people are accustomed to is broken up in three ways: a piece of meat, some kind of starch (typically white potatoes or rice), and an overcooked veggie. This "pie plate" concept goes out the window on a plant-based diet. Instead, think of your plate or bowl as having so much variety, texture, and color that exact portions or amounts don't really matter.

I'll break this down a bit further. When thinking of dinner from now on, don't think of foods as their own sections of the plate; they may be layered together in a pot or casserole dish instead. Or maybe you have just two things on your plate, such as a quinoa salad and a homemade veggie burger, which can be combined and eaten together. Or a plate may be made up of mostly carbohydrates that together make a perfect plant protein. Also, many lunch items can be served for dinner, and vice versa.

In time, you'll discover so much more variety when you make the switch to plants. Your dinners become colorful and dazzling sensations that you'll love.

If you have kids or (ahem) picky adults in the family, try these tips for keeping their minds and tummies happy:

- ✔ Get them involved in the process to add their own flair to pasta or pick what veggies go into the stir-fry.

- ✔ Let them help with age-appropriate prep work.

- ✔ Always have their favorite veggies and grains available at dinner — either as a stand-alone dish or as an ingredient in new dishes to encourage them to try new things.

- ✔ Introduce new items slowly. Don't unleash a seven-course meal of dishes they've never had. Make sure a new addition is just one part of a dinner that's full of familiar foods.

Zesty Pesto Pasta with White Beans

Prep time: 5 min • **Cook time:** 20 min • **Yield:** 10 servings

Ingredients	*Directions*
Sea salt	*1* Boil a large pot of water, add sea salt, and cook the pasta until al dente or tender, about 7 to 10 minutes. Drain, but keep the pasta in the pot.
One 16-ounce package whole-grain pasta, such as kamut pasta or brown rice pasta	
Pesto Sauce (see the following recipe)	*2* On low to medium heat, add the pesto to the cooked pasta; add the beans and spinach. Stir until well combined and the spinach has wilted.
1 tablespoon olive oil	
2 cups spinach or Swiss chard	*3* Place a few ladles of the pasta into a bowl and serve alongside a salad or a bowl of minestrone soup.
1 cup cooked white beans	

Pesto Sauce

¼ cup pine nuts or walnuts, toasted	*1* Grind the nuts in a food processor until you get a paste.
2 cups fresh basil	
¼ cup olive oil	*2* Add the remaining ingredients and process for a few minutes until well combined.
1 to 2 cloves garlic	
2 tablespoons fresh lemon juice	
1 teaspoon white miso	
1 tablespoon honey	
salt and pepper to taste	

Per serving: Calories 279 (From Fat 90); Fat 10g (Saturated 1g); Cholesterol 0mg; Sodium 28mg; Carbohydrate 40g (Dietary Fiber 6g); Protein 8g.

Note: Gluten-free pasta, like brown-rice pasta, often takes about 15 minutes to cook.

Tip: For perfect pasta every time, bring your pot of water to a boil. Add the pasta, bring the water back up to a boil, cover, turn off the heat, and let stand for 12 to 15 minutes. Don't touch or stir your pasta, and it will be perfectly cooked!

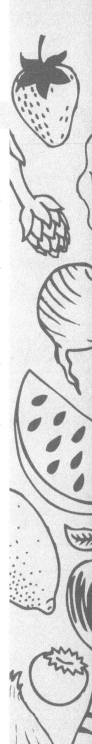

Quinoa with Chickpeas and Spinach

Prep time: 15 min • **Cook time:** 25 min • **Yield:** 8 servings

Ingredients	*Directions*
1 cup water	*1* Combine the water and orange juice in a saucepan and bring to a boil. Add the salt, orange zest, and quinoa and return to a boil.
¾ cup fresh-squeezed orange juice	
½ teaspoon sea salt	*2* Reduce the heat, cover, and simmer for 12 minutes, or until all the liquid is absorbed.
zest from 1 organic orange, approximately ½ tablespoon	
1 cup quinoa, rinsed and drained	*3* Remove the quinoa from the heat, keep it covered, and let sit for 3 minutes.
1 tablespoon extra virgin olive oil	*4* While the quinoa is cooking, heat the oil in a large skillet that has a tight-fitting lid. Add the onions and sauté over medium heat for about 5 minutes, until they have softened and begun to brown. Add the garlic and sauté until golden.
1 medium onion, chopped	
3 garlic cloves, minced	
½ cup organic raisins	
1 cup cooked chickpeas or organic canned chickpeas	*5* Add the raisins, chickpeas, and spinach. Cover and cook over medium heat for 3 minutes, or just until the spinach has wilted. Adjust the heat if necessary.
1 to 2 cups spinach leaves, trimmed, washed, drained, and dried	
salt to taste	*6* Drain any excess water and season to taste with salt.
½ teaspoon cinnamon	*7* To serve, fold the vegetables into the quinoa. Stir in the cinnamon. Squeeze some orange juice over the quinoa. Garnish with toasted pine nuts and orange wedges.
¼ cup toasted pine nuts or almonds	
1 orange, cut into wedges	

Per serving: Calories 198 (From Fat 63); Fat 7g (Saturated 0.5g); Cholesterol 0mg; Sodium 173mg; Carbohydrate 31g (Dietary Fiber 4g); Protein 6g.

Hearty Vegetable Cacciatore

Prep time: 15 min • **Cook time:** 18–30 min • **Yield:** 6 servings

Ingredients	Directions
2 tablespoons olive oil	*1* Heat the oil in a large saucepan and cook the garlic and leeks over medium heat until soft.
2 cloves garlic, minced	
1 cup diced leeks or diced onions	*2* Add the remaining ingredients.
1 cup diced carrots	
1 cup diced celery	*3* Cook for 15 to 30 minutes until the moisture has evaporated and the dish is reduced and thickened. Remove the bay leaves.
3 cups sliced mushrooms	
½ cup finely chopped fresh basil, or 1 teaspoon dried basil	*4* Serve with whole-grain or gluten-free pasta, brown rice, or quinoa, or enjoy it on its own.
2 tablespoons fresh oregano, or 1 teaspoon dried oregano	
3 bay leaves	
2 cups tomato sauce	
1 teaspoon salt	
½ cup finely chopped parsley	
1 to 2 cups cubed organic tofu	

Per serving: Calories 147 (From Fat 72); Fat 8g (Saturated 1.5g); Cholesterol 0mg; Sodium 858mg; Carbohydrate 12g (Dietary Fiber 4g); Protein 9g.

Vary It! Instead of organic tofu, opt for white beans, chickpeas, or fava beans for a hearty vegetarian source of protein. Or use this as a sauce to top the Mushroom and Chickpea Loaf (see the recipe later in this chapter).

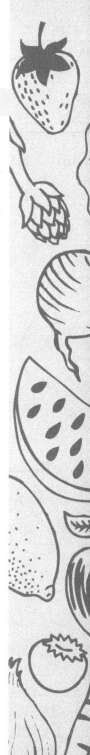

Black Bean Cumin Burgers

Prep time: 15 min, plus soaking time • **Cook time:** 40 min • **Yield:** 8–12 servings

Ingredients	*Directions*
1 cup black beans, soaked overnight and rinsed, or 2 cans organic black beans, drained and rinsed	*1* Preheat the oven to 350 degrees, and line a baking sheet with parchment paper.
1 cup grated sweet potatoes	*2* Place the soaked beans in a pot with water (cover the beans by 1 to 2 inches). Bring the water and beans to a boil. Lower the heat and simmer for 1½ hours. Remove from the heat and drain.
½ cup almond butter	
½ cup diced red onion	*3* Place the beans in a bowl and mash. Stir in the remaining ingredients.
¼ cup brown-rice flour	
2 tablespoons tamari	*4* Scoop ⅓ cup of the batter to form a burger patty and place on the baking sheet. Continue until all the batter is used.
3 cloves garlic, minced	
1 tablespoon cumin	
	5 Bake for 30 minutes until golden brown.

Per serving: *Calories 217 (From Fat 81); Fat 9g (Saturated 1g); Cholesterol 0mg; Sodium 405mg; Carbohydrate 26g (Dietary Fiber 7g); Protein 9g.*

Vary It! For a nut-free option, use sunflower-seed butter instead of almond butter.

Tip: Enjoy this burger on a sprouted-grain bun or wrap, with brown rice or quinoa, or on a salad for a complete dinner. You may want to add some salsa or avocado for a tasty topping.

Cooking with oils: What to use and when

The world of oil is a mysterious, liquidy place. Understanding it isn't as hard as it seems, though, and understanding which ones should be used greatly enhances recipes and cooking techniques. Here's a quick rundown of which oils to use in which circumstances.

✔ On low to medium heat, try olive, sunflower, safflower, or sesame oils.

✔ If a recipe calls for high heat, go with coconut oil or grapeseed oil.

✔ When no heat is required as in raw recipes, olive, flax, chia, or hemp oils are the best. **Note:** These oils *should never* be used with heat. Olive oil is the only oil that can withstand low-temperature heating.

When certain oils are heated beyond their smoke point (which means they start smoking in the pan), they are no long stable and become toxic to the body. Be mindful of which oil you're using at which temperature.

Arame Soba Noodle Salad

Prep time: 15 min • **Cook time:** 15 min • **Yield:** 6 servings

Ingredients	*Directions*
6 cups water	*1* Bring 5 cups of water to a boil in a large pot. Add the basil, rosemary, and salt.
1 teaspoon dried basil	
½ teaspoon dried rosemary	*2* Add the noodles, cook until al dente (8 to 10 minutes), rinse, and drain.
½ teaspoon salt	
8 ounces kamut or buckwheat soba noodles	*3* In a separate dish, soak the arame in 1 cup of cold water for about 10 minutes, then drain.
½ cup arame (sea vegetable)	
2 cloves garlic, crushed	*4* In a large bowl, whisk together the garlic, ginger, vinegar, sesame oil, and tamari.
1 teaspoon gingerroot, grated	
¼ cup rice vinegar	*5* Add the warm noodles to the sauce and toss to coat. Let the noodles sit and absorb the sauce for 10 minutes to 1 hour.
¼ cup toasted sesame oil	
3 tablespoons tamari	
1 cup organic edamame, shelled and cooked (optional)	*6* Stir in the edamame, carrots, onions, and arame.
1 carrot, grated	*7* Serve in small bowls and sprinkle with toasted pine nuts or sesame seeds.
1 cup chopped green onions	
½ cup toasted pine nuts or black sesame seeds	

Per serving: Calories 341 (From Fat 171); Fat 19g (Saturated 2g); Cholesterol 0mg; Sodium 735mg; Carbohydrate 36g (Dietary Fiber 4g); Protein 10g.

Note: Enjoy this dish with a side of steamed greens. Add a dollop of tahini to make this salad extra creamy.

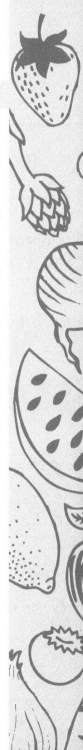

Warm Festive Farro Salad

Prep time: 15 min • **Cook time:** 60 min • **Yield:** 6 servings

Ingredients	*Directions*
1 cup farro (spelt), soaked overnight in enough water to cover it completely	*1* Preheat the oven to 350 degrees.
½ butternut squash, peeled and cubed	*2* Rinse the farro and place it in a pot with 1 cup of water. Bring to a boil, reduce the heat, and simmer 30 to 45 minutes. Set aside the cooked farro.
¼ cup olive oil, plus 2 tablespoons, divided	
1 clove garlic, minced	*3* While the farro is cooking, place the butternut squash on a baking tray and toss with 1 tablespoon of olive oil and bake for 30 minutes.
1 red onion, chopped	
1 cup portobello mushrooms, chopped	*4* In a skillet, heat 1 tablespoon of olive oil with the garlic over medium heat and add the onions, mushrooms, and currants; sauté until softened.
⅓ cup currants or dried cranberries	
1 cup thinly sliced rainbow chard or spinach	*5* Add the chard, sea salt, dry herbs, and balsamic vinegar. Let sit for a few minutes to let the flavors combine and the chard wilt.
1 teaspoon sea salt	
1 teaspoon oregano	*6* Place the cooked farro in a large bowl and add 2 to 4 tablespoons of olive oil to taste. Add the butternut squash and the onion, mushroom, and chard mixture. Stir to combine. Top with walnuts.
dash of herbes de Provence	
3 tablespoons balsamic vinegar	
¼ cup toasted walnuts, or pine nuts	

Per serving: Calories 306 (From Fat 153); Fat 17g (Saturated 2g); Cholesterol 0mg; Sodium 251mg; Carbohydrate 31g (Dietary Fiber 4g); Protein 6g.

Vary It! For an extra dose of protein, add 1 cup of cooked white beans at the end of Step 6. This gives this dish a richer texture.

Sweet Potato Shepherd's Pie

Prep time: 30 min • **Cook time:** 45 min • **Yield:** 10 servings

Ingredients	Directions
2 teaspoons extra-virgin olive oil	*1* Preheat the oven to 350 degrees.
1 clove garlic, peeled and crushed	*2* Heat ¼ cup water and olive oil in a large saucepan. Add the garlic, onion, sea salt, celery, and bay leaf and simmer for about 3 minutes.
1 onion, peeled and sliced	
1 teaspoon sea salt	
2 sticks celery, washed and chopped	*3* Add the squash and heat for another 3 minutes, stirring. Pour in 2 cups of water and bring to a boil over medium heat. Simmer gently for 10 minutes, stirring occasionally.
1 bay leaf	
1 to 2 cups butternut squash, peeled, halved, deseeded, and cut into small pieces	*4* Add the kidney beans, cauliflower, zucchini, broccoli, and carrots. Simmer for another 5 minutes until the squash is just tender. Stir in the parsley and arrowroot. Transfer to a large baking dish or 2 small baking dishes greased with grapeseed oil.
2 cups cooked kidney beans, or 1 can or organic kidney beans	
½ head cauliflower, cut into slices or chopped	*5* Mix the sweet potato mash with a little of the steamed cooking water in a small bowl. Add a dash of tamari.
2 medium zucchini, sliced	
½ head broccoli, finely chopped	*6* Using a fork or the back of a spoon, spread the sweet potato mixture over the vegetable mixture. Bake at 350 degrees for 15 to 20 minutes, or until the pie is set.
3 medium carrots, sliced	
2 tablespoons finely chopped fresh parsley	*7* To serve, scoop out a large square of the pie and serve with a side of cooked millet, brown rice, or quinoa and some steamed green leafy vegetables like kale.
1 teaspoon arrowroot	
4 sweet potatoes, steamed for 15 minutes until soft, and mashed (reserve a small amount of cooking water)	
dash of tamari	

Per serving: *Calories 152 (From Fat 12); Fat 1.5g (Saturated 0g); Cholesterol 0mg; Sodium 238mg; Carbohydrate 31g (Dietary Fiber 7g); Protein 6g.*

Tip: To give this dish more flavor, add a few spoonsful of the Tahini-Miso Gravy; find the recipe in Chapter 15.

Tangy Tempeh Teriyaki Stir-Fry

Prep time: 15 min • **Cook time:** 15 min • **Yield:** 8 servings

Ingredients	Directions
Marinade (see the following recipe)	*1* Cut the tempeh or tofu into small cubes.
10.5-ounce package of organic tempeh or tofu	*2* In a medium saucepan or wok, combine the tempeh or tofu with ¾ of the marinade, along with the onions, carrots, and celery. Cover and simmer over medium heat for 5 to 10 minutes.
1 onion, chopped	
1 cup chopped carrots	
1 cup chopped celery	*3* Place the broccoli in the wok and cook until just tender.
1 head (about 2 cups) broccoli or cauliflower, cut into florets	*4* Combine the bok choy with the tempeh or tofu and stir with the remaining marinade until the bok choy softens a bit.
1 head (about 2 cups) bok choy, chopped	
¼ cup sesame seeds	*5* Make sure everything is well coated. Top with sesame seeds and serve with brown rice, soba noodles, or quinoa.

Marinade

2 tablespoons toasted
sesame oil

¼ cup tamari

1 to 2 cloves garlic, minced

1 tablespoon minced ginger

juice of 1 orange

1 to 2 tablespoons brown-rice
vinegar

1 tablespoon brown-rice syrup

1 In a bowl, combine the marinade ingredients and set aside.

Per serving: Calories 129 (From Fat 63); Fat 7g (Saturated 1g); Cholesterol 0mg; Sodium 551mg; Carbohydrate 11g (Dietary Fiber 3g); Protein 6g.

Tip: For extra flavor, marinate the tempeh cubes in half of the marinade for up to an hour before making this dish to allow the flavors to absorb.

Note: Be sure not to overcook your green veggies — you want them to remain green. The goal is to keep them crisp and tender. Add them at the end and let them cook down with the warmth of the stir-fry.

Vary It! Try this stir-fry with different veggies that are in season. Peppers, asparagus, and Japanese eggplant can all be swapped in to make different variations.

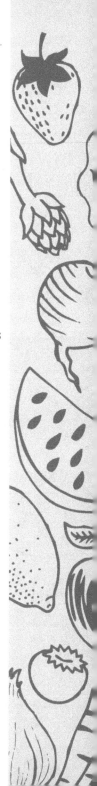

Mushroom and Chickpea Loaf

Prep time: 20 min, plus bean soaking and cooking time • **Cook time:** 55 min • **Yield:** 6–8 servings

Ingredients	Directions
2 tablespoons grapeseed oil	*1* Preheat the oven to 350 degrees.
2 teaspoons minced garlic	
1 cup chopped onions	*2* In a large sauté pan, heat the oil over medium-high heat.
2 medium carrots, chopped	
½ cup chopped zucchini	*3* Add the garlic, onions, and carrots; cook for 4 minutes.
1 cup chopped mushrooms	
1½ cups chickpeas (soaked overnight and cooked), or one 14-ounce can of organic chickpeas	*4* Stir in the zucchini and mushrooms and sauté for 8 minutes, or until softened.
1½ cups cooked white beans	*5* In a food processor, combine the zucchini mixture and the remaining ingredients.
⅓ cup dried wheat-free bread crumbs	
¼ cup organic tomato sauce	*6* Pulse on and off until the mixture is finely chopped and well combined. Press into a loaf pan greased with grapeseed oil.
2 tablespoons nutritional yeast	
1 tablespoon arrowroot powder	
1 tablespoon Dijon mustard	*7* Bake uncovered for about 40 minutes.
½ cup whole rolled oats	*8* Allow the loaf to set for approximately 20 minutes to cool. Remove from the pan and slice into 8–10 slices.
¼ teaspoon ground pepper	
1 teaspoon dried basil	
¼ teaspoon cumin	*9* Serve with the Hearty Vegetable Cacciatore (see the recipe earlier in this chapter), Tahini-Miso Gravy in Chapter 15, or extra tomato sauce.
1 teaspoon oregano	
1 tablespoon tamari	

Per serving: Calories 174 (From Fat 54); Fat 6g (Saturated 0.5g); Cholesterol 0mg; Sodium 414mg; Carbohydrate 25g (Dietary Fiber 6g); Protein 7g.

Note: Dried chickpeas need to cook for 1½ to 2 hours, and dried white beans need to cook for 45 to 60 minutes.

Chapter 13

Guiltless Desserts

In This Chapter

▶ Understanding different sweeteners you can use for baking

▶ Getting to know alternatives to eggs, dairy, and wheat

▶ Discovering delicious dessert recipes that will make your mouth water

*I*f we didn't have desserts, the world would be a very sad place. Sometimes it seems we may be heading in that direction: People feel guilty after consuming a well-deserved delicious treat, or they don't consume desserts at all for fear of gaining weight or experiencing other negative health conditions. It's true that there is a lot of junk out there, so you have to be discerning. This chapter proves that you can enjoy every bite of your dessert — as long as you eat it in moderation and it's made with wholesome, plant-based ingredients.

Concerned about taste and satisfaction? You're not alone, but you needn't worry. Plant-based desserts are loaded with fiber, minerals, and vitamins that actually fill you up, so you're not as tempted to eat that whole cake in one sitting (bye-bye, guilt), *and* they're just as yummy!

Getting to Know Alternative Sweeteners

Sugar is sugar in any form, so you need to watch your intake of alternative sweeteners, even if they're plant-based. Be sure to eat your treats in moderation and with a conscious mind. That said, using sweetening agents that aren't as refined as white sugar is a key to healthy baking and tasty desserts, so get to know the ones you should start stocking in your pantry pronto:

▶ **The liquids:** Maple syrup, honey, coconut nectar, date syrup, molasses, agave, and brown-rice syrup. You can use these in place of regular sugar in most recipes, especially beverages. Experiment and see which flavors you like best.

Agave has substantial drawbacks, including a high fructose content. Some health experts even consider it worse for your health than high fructose corn syrup, so use it sparingly or not at all.

✔ **The granules and crystals:** Maple sugar, coconut sugar, sucanat, and organic cane sugar. These are all amazing in baked recipes, such as brownies, muffins, cakes, and cookies.

✔ **Low glycemic:** Stevia, xylitol, and lakanto. These are great for people with blood-sugar disorders such as diabetes. They are easy to use; however, they can produce an overpowering flavor, especially when baking, so use them sparingly.

Be sure to look for green powdered stevia. Stevia is a plant leaf, so any white or liquid derivative is an overprocessed version. Keeping the leaf as whole as possible is better for you. When you use stevia, add it in very small increments because it's overpoweringly sweet. A little bit goes a long way.

Xylitol is not well absorbed in the intestines; it draws water into the colon and can have a laxative effect.

✔ **Fruits:** Dates, bananas, apples, figs, lacuma, and dried fruit. These can be used to sweeten baked goods, breakfast porridge, and smoothies. They contain naturally occurring sugars and have the added benefit of fiber, vitamins, and minerals. Depending on the recipe, you may want to use these wholesome and natural sources of sugar.

You may never have heard of lacuma. Lacuma is a fruit that is low glycemic and contains many minerals and beta carotene. It has a sweet maple flavor and can be used cup for cup as a replacement for sugar.

To make dates into a liquid consistency, cover approximately ½ cup of dates with water and soak them overnight or in warm water for an hour and then puree in a high-speed blender. After you have a paste, you can then use it in place of sugar as a liquid ingredient.

Artificial sweeteners, like the ones in those little colored packets at restaurants, are chemically derived and toxic to your health. Eliminate these completely from your diet.

You don't have to follow too many rules in terms of which sweeteners to use in which circumstance; you can use different types of sweeteners in various recipes. The real fun is in getting creative and experimenting, but here are some general match-ups to get you started:

✔ **Light cakes and muffins:** Maple syrup is a great go-to for these.

✔ **Dark cakes, brownies, and dessert squares:** These desserts work best with richer sugars like sucanat and coconut sugar.

What's up, honey?

Honey is a complicated topic, especially from a vegan's perspective. Many believe that because honey is sourced from an animal, it's not a plant-based food. Technically, however, it's derived from a plant, and the process of making honey can certainly be ethical, as long as the bees aren't harmed in the process.

I suggest that people make their own decision about what feels right for them. Choosing a local, organic, raw, or unpasteurized form of honey is,

I believe, a healthy part of even a plant-based diet. However, other alternatives are available, so don't fret — you have plenty to choose from if you don't want to use honey. Because honey is a living food, it offers a slew of health benefits that other sweeteners don't, such as antiviral and antibacterial properties.

- ✔ **Granola and cookies:** Use maple syrup, maple sugar, or coconut sugar.
- ✔ **Raw desserts, creams, and puddings:** Honey, coconut nectar, or maple syrup and dates are the way to go.

When substituting a liquid sugar for a granulated one, make sure to use ¼ cup less. For example, 1 cup of white sugar = ¾ cup of maple syrup.

No Eggs, No Dairy, No Problem!

It may seem strange to make a dessert without traditional ingredients such as eggs and dairy products; however, plant-based desserts actually work quite well without butter, cream, milk, or eggs. You can use many natural substitutions.

It's easier to bake in the plant-based world than it is in the non-plant-based world because plant-based baking is so much more forgiving. When you make a plant-based dessert, you have a little more room for error; you don't have to make exact measurements like you do with a traditional recipe for baked goods. A plant-based recipe is usually a wet-and-dry mix as opposed to getting the measurements and timing exactly right. Some people are fearful of baking for this reason.

However, if you're attempting something more technical and specialized, such as complex fancy birthday cakes, pies, or pastries, that's a different conversation altogether, and I don't get into that here. For the sake of this book, I keep the desserts rather simple, focusing on innovative plant-based ingredients that everyone can use and will love to eat!

Here's a quick rundown on how to make general substitutions for the foundation ingredients in the dessert world:

- ✔ **Eggs:** To replace one egg, mix 1 tablespoon of ground flax or ground chia seeds with 3 tablespoons of water.

- ✔ **Milk:** Rice milk, almond milk, coconut milk, and hempseed milk can replace dairy milk, measure for measure.

- ✔ **Butter:** Coconut oil, grapeseed oil, and sunflower oil can replace this, measure for measure.

- ✔ **Buttermilk:** To produce a replacement, combine 1 cup of alternative milk with 1 tablespoon of apple-cider vinegar.

- ✔ **Cream:** Try using coconut milk or cashew milk as a measure-for-measure replacement.

Praise for coconut oil

I make wonderful recipes with coconut oil — it is one of my favorite ingredients. It is dairy-free, gluten-free, and full of delicious flavor. It can also be heated to high temperatures in baking and stir-frying and used raw in smoothies and desserts.

These days, coconut oil is one of the most controversial ingredients. The media and medical practitioners say it's unhealthy, fattening, and damaging to the arteries. In reality, it's only the hydrogenated version of coconut oil that's bad for you.

Many studies have documented the health benefits of virgin coconut oil (in its original state): It's antibacterial, antiviral, and energizing, and

it has healing properties. The medium-chain triglycerides found in coconut oil help people with digestive problems, infections, and low metabolism. It boosts energy and even protects against serious health problems, such as cancer and diabetes.

As a bonus, you can drink the water straight from the coconut and use it as an energy drink before, after, or during exercise. So don't be afraid of this wonderful and tasty fruit: Use it whole, use its water, use its butter, and use its shell. There are endless possibilities!

Apricot Fig Oat Bars

Prep time: 10 min • **Cook time:** 35 min • **Yield:** 12 servings

Ingredients	Directions
1 cup chopped unsulphured dried apricots (brown)	*1* Preheat the oven to 350 degrees.
1 cup chopped dried figs	*2* In a saucepan, combine the apricots, figs, orange juice, and water. Cover and cook on low heat for 10 minutes, stirring occasionally. Remove from the heat and set aside.
Juice of 1 orange or 1 lemon	
½ cup water	
½ cup coconut oil	*3* In a large bowl, cream together the coconut oil and sucanat. Stir in the flour, salt, and baking soda. Add the oats and mix using your hands. The dough will be crumbly but will hold together when squeezed.
½ cup sucanat or maple sugar or coconut sugar	
1¾ cups light spelt flour	
¼ teaspoon sea salt	*4* Press ⅔ of the dough into an 8- or 9-inch square baking pan greased with coconut oil.
½ teaspoon baking soda	
1 cup rolled oats	*5* Stir the apricot mixture and spread it over the dough. Crumble the remaining dough on top.
	6 Bake for 30 minutes. Cut into bars after the pan has cooled completely.

Per serving: *Calories 252 (From Fat 90); Fat 10g (Saturated 8g); Cholesterol 0mg; Sodium 89mg; Carbohydrate 37g (Dietary Fiber 4g); Protein 4g.*

Tip: The best way to cut these into clean squares, especially for serving, is to allow the pan to cool completely, refrigerate it for a few hours or overnight, and then cut the dessert into squares.

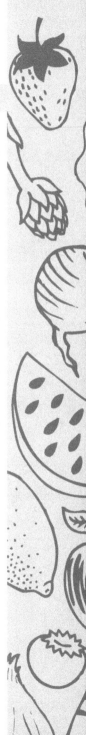

Carob Fig Frozen Fudge

Prep time: 10 min, plus soaking and freezing time • **Yield:** 12 servings

Ingredients	Directions
1 cup figs	*1* Place the figs in a bowl, cover with water, and soak for about an hour, until soft. Drain, reserving the liquid.
1½ cups water	
1 tablespoon pure vanilla	*2* In a blender, blend the figs and vanilla until smooth, slowly adding the water from the figs, as needed, to form a creamy consistency.
½ to 1 cup almond butter or sunflower butter	
½ to 1 cup raw carob powder	*3* Transfer the fig mixture into a large bowl, add the almond butter, and stir to combine.
½ cup hempseeds	
	4 In a separate bowl, mix the carob powder and hempseeds.
	5 Gradually add the dry carob mixture into the wet fig mixture. Stir well.
	6 Press evenly into an 8-x-8-inch baking pan and freeze until firm (about 3 hours).
	7 To serve, cut into 1-inch squares.

Per serving: Calories 115 (From Fat 45); Fat 5g (Saturated 0.5g); Cholesterol 0mg; Sodium 8mg; Carbohydrate 12g (Dietary Fiber 3g); Protein 4g.

Vary It! You can roll this mixture into bite-size balls instead of squares for little fudge bites on the go.

Jam Dot Cookies

Prep time: 20 min • **Cook time:** 15–20 min • **Yield:** 20 cookies

Ingredients	Directions
1 cup ground almonds	**1** Preheat the oven to 350 degrees. Line two baking sheets with parchment paper.
2 cups light spelt flour	
¼ teaspoon ground cinnamon	**2** In a medium bowl, combine the almonds, flour, and cinnamon. Mix well to combine.
½ cup melted coconut oil	
½ cup maple syrup	**3** In a separate bowl, blend the oil, maple syrup, and sea salt. Add to the flour mixture and stir to combine.
pinch of sea salt	
1 jar of "no sugar added" raspberry or apricot jam	**4** Roll into walnut-sized balls. Place on the baking sheets and press down with your thumb.
	5 Fill the indentations with jam and bake for 15 to 20 minutes.

Per serving: Calories 154 (From Fat 72); Fat 8g (Saturated 4.5g); Cholesterol 0mg; Sodium 1mg; Carbohydrate 19g (Dietary Fiber 2g); Protein 2g.

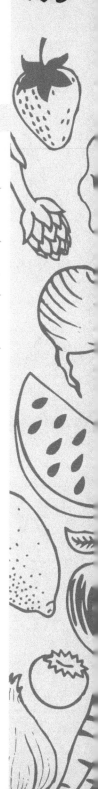

Chewy Oatmeal Raisin Cookies

Prep time: 10 min • **Cook time:** 12–14 min • **Yield:** 24 servings

Ingredients	Directions
¾ cup spelt flour	**1** Preheat the oven to 350 degrees. Line two cookie sheets with parchment paper.
½ teaspoon baking soda	
½ scant teaspoon salt	**2** Mix together the flour, baking soda, salt, and cinnamon. Set aside.
½ teaspoon cinnamon	
½ cup sucanat or maple sugar	**3** Mix the sugars, maple syrup, applesauce, oil, and vanilla together in a medium bowl. Add the flour mixture and stir until blended.
¼ cup coconut sugar	
2 tablespoons maple syrup	
¼ cup applesauce	**4** Stir in the oats, followed by the raisins. Let sit for 10 minutes.
¼ cup melted coconut oil	
½ teaspoon vanilla	**5** Drop by rounded teaspoonful onto the cookie sheets about 1 inch apart. Bake for 12 to 14 minutes. Let cool for 2 to 5 minutes on the cookie sheets, then carefully use a spatula to transfer the cookies onto a wire rack.
1½ cups rolled oats	
½ cup raisins	

Per serving: Calories 92 (From Fat 27); Fat 3g (Saturated 2g); Cholesterol 0mg; Sodium 76mg; Carbohydrate 15g (Dietary Fiber 1); Protein 1g.

Tip: You can use just one type of granulated sweetener if desired — sucanat, maple, or coconut. I provide the option of a few for variety, but the recipe works fine with ¾ cup of just one of them.

Amazing Banana Bread

Prep time: 10 min • **Cook time:** 20–40 min • **Yield:** 8–12 servings

Ingredients	Directions
⅓ cup applesauce	*1* Preheat the oven to 350 degrees. Either grease a loaf pan with coconut oil or line two 12-cup muffin tins with parchment paper cups.
1 tablespoon ground flaxseeds	
2 to 4 ripe bananas (depending on their size), peeled	*2* Mix the applesauce and flaxseeds together in a bowl. Allow to set for 2 minutes.
½ cup rice milk	
¼ cup coconut oil, melted, or grapeseed oil	*3* Mix the bananas, rice milk, oil, and maple syrup into the applesauce. Set aside.
¼ cup maple syrup	
2 cups organic spelt flour	*4* Combine the flour, baking soda, baking powder, cinnamon, and salt in a large bowl. Then fold the wet ingredients into the dry ingredients slowly. Mix until there are no lumps. Stir in the blueberries or chocolate chips.
1 teaspoon baking soda	
1 teaspoon baking powder	
¼ teaspoon cinnamon	
½ teaspoon sea salt	*5* Drop by spoonsful into the prepared muffin tins or pour the batter into the loaf pan.
1 cup blueberries or dairy-free dark chocolate chips	
	6 Bake for 20 minutes for muffins or 30 to 40 minutes for a loaf.

Per serving: Calories 166 (From Fat 54); Fat 6g (Saturated 4g); Cholesterol 0mg; Sodium 243mg; Carbohydrate 28g (Dietary Fiber 3g); Protein 3g.

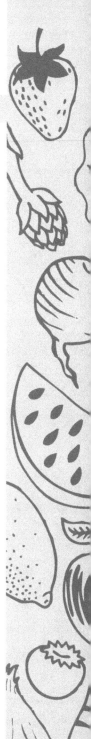

Chocolate Avocado Pudding

Prep time: 5 min, plus soaking time • **Yield:** 2+ servings

Ingredients	Directions
2 ripe avocados, peeled and cut into small pieces	**1** Combine all the ingredients except those used for the garnish in a blender and whirl on high until well blended into a thick, creamy pudding.
1 tablespoon vanilla extract	
2 to 4 tablespoons maple syrup	**2** Divide the pudding into two or more servings.
5 Medjool dates (soaked overnight or in warm water for 20 to 30 minutes)	**3** Top with the cacao nibs, coconut flakes, or raspberries.
2 tablespoons pure, unsweetened cacao powder	
1 to 2 tablespoons almond butter, coconut butter, or other seed-based butter	
1 ripe banana, peeled	
1 teaspoon cinnamon	
Cacao nibs, coconut flakes, or raspberries for garnish	

Per serving: Calories 662 (From Fat 270); Fat 30g (Saturated 4g); Cholesterol 0mg; Sodium 56mg; Carbohydrate 98g (Dietary Fiber 18g); Protein 9g.

Brown Rice Pudding

Prep time: 15 min, plus cooling time • **Cook time:** 60 min • **Yield:** 10 servings

Ingredients	Directions
1½ cups brown rice	*1* Preheat the oven to 350 degrees.
3 cups water	
2 tablespoons arrowroot powder	*2* Bring the brown rice and water to a boil in a heavy, medium saucepan.
1½ cups vanilla rice milk, divided	*3* Reduce the heat to low, cover, and simmer for 40 to 50 minutes, or until very soft.
¼ cup raisins	
¼ cup maple syrup	*4* In a large bowl, dissolve the arrowroot powder in 1 cup of milk. Then add the cooked rice, raisins, maple syrup, vanilla, cinnamon, and salt, and mix well to combine.
1 teaspoon vanilla powder or vanilla extract	
1 tablespoon ground cinnamon, or 2 cinnamon sticks	
½ teaspoon sea salt	*5* Transfer to a large baking dish greased with coconut oil. Cover with foil and bake for 1 hour, or until browned and bubbly.
1 teaspoon pistachios	
1 teaspoon almonds	*6* Remove from the oven and stir in the remaining ½ cup of rice milk. Let cool for about 1 hour before serving. Garnish with pistachios and almonds.

Per serving: Calories 161 (From Fat 9); Fat 1g (Saturated 0g); Cholesterol 0mg; Sodium 120mg; Carbohydrate 34g (Dietary Fiber 1.5g); Protein 2.5g.

Note: If you use cinnamon sticks, remember to fish them out at the end so you don't crunch down on one.

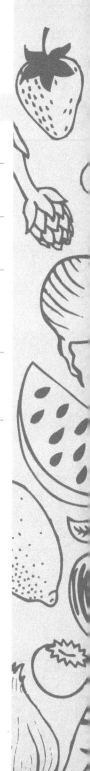

Carrot Pineapple Layer Cake

Prep time: 15 min • **Cook time:** 40 min • **Yield:** 10 servings

Ingredients	Directions
Cashew Cream (see the following recipe)	**1** Preheat the oven to 350 degrees.
½ cup grapeseed oil or sunflower oil	**2** In a medium bowl, mix together the grapeseed oil, maple syrup, apple-cider vinegar, rice milk, and vanilla for about 2 minutes. Add the carrot, pineapple, and coconut and stir until combined. Set aside.
1 cup maple syrup	
2 teaspoons apple-cider vinegar	
¼ cup rice milk	**3** In a large bowl, combine the flour, salt, cinnamon, baking powder, and walnuts. Make a well in the center of these dry ingredients and pour the wet ingredients into the well. Stir gently until all the ingredients are combined thoroughly.
1 teaspoon vanilla	
1 cup grated carrot	
1 cup chopped pineapple, canned crushed (and drained), or fresh	**4** Scoop the mixture into two 9-inch round pans greased with grapeseed oil and dusted with spelt flour.
½ cup dried unsweetened coconut flakes	**5** Bake for 40 minutes. Poke a toothpick, fork, or skewer into the center of the cake to make sure it's done; the toothpick should come out clean.
1½ cups light spelt flour	
¼ teaspoon sea salt	**6** Once cool, run a knife around the inside edge of the pans to loosen the cake from the sides. Turn them onto plates.
½ teaspoon cinnamon	
1 teaspoon baking powder	
½ cup chopped walnuts	**7** Spread cashew cream on top of the bottom cake, add the top cake, and continue to spread the remaining cream over the top and sides.
Walnuts, chopped pineapple, or coconut flakes for garnish	
	8 Garnish with walnuts, chopped pineapple, or coconut flakes.

Cashew Cream

1 to 2 cups cashews (soaked overnight in 1 to 2 cups water and drained)

1 tablespoon almond butter or coconut butter

2 tablespoons brown-rice syrup

1 teaspoon cinnamon

1 teaspoon maple syrup (optional)

1 Place all the ingredients in a food processor and blend until well combined and creamy.

Per serving: *Calories 476 (From Fat 261); Fat 29g (Saturated 5.5g); Cholesterol 0mg; Sodium 127mg; Carbohydrate 49g (Dietary Fiber 4.5g); Protein 7g.*

Note: Make sure you let the cakes cool thoroughly on a rack before attempting to remove them from the pans (otherwise, they may stick because of the pineapple).

Note: This cake has a wet, thick consistency from the pineapple, carrot, and coconut. Don't expect this to be your typical dry carrot cake; you'll be pleasantly surprised.

Tip: The cashew cream makes an absolutely yummy addition to fruit salad!

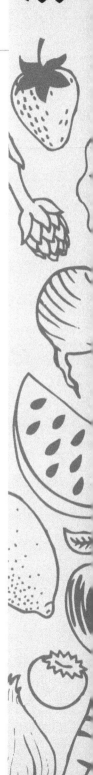

Chapter 14

Sensational Snacks

*L*ong gone are the days of three square meals; in today's go-go-go world, this just isn't realistic anymore. We are more mobile and more active, and we have to cram more into our days than ever before, which means we need more fuel to keep us going. Plus — let's be honest — we all love to snack! The goal for a "snacker" — or, shall I say, regular eater — is to reach for good foods that make you feel good, not junk foods that make you feel bad. The good news is that you have plenty of friendly plant-based options from which to choose.

In this chapter, I explain how snacking is beneficial to your health and how to balance the flavors your body craves. Then I provide all sorts of recipes that will satisfy your hunger when you just want a quick bite.

Boosting Your Metabolism with Healthy Snacking

An old adage says that the more often you eat, the faster your metabolism functions. Although a lot of metabolism is genetics, you can influence it by how frequently you eat. When you wait a long time between meals, your metabolism actually slows down to conserve your body's remaining fuel and energy. When you constantly eat throughout the day, it stays in high gear. Why does this matter? Well, having a faster (or higher) metabolism means you can turn your food into energy and burn your energy efficiently and quickly. When your metabolism slows down, the calories are slower to burn away and ultimately can turn into extra weight. Snacks keep the furnace burning.

To boost your metabolism, you need to have regular snacks in addition to your three meals. So you may eat upwards of five times a day, depending on your metabolism, appetite, and activity levels.

When you think of the average snack, chances are you envision one favorite item — a bag of pretzels or perhaps a cookie, or maybe you're one of the good ones and reach for an apple! But your snack probably isn't as powerful as it could be, even if you do reach for the apple. The key is to make the snack a little more complex than just an apple, especially on a plant-based diet.

Snacks should be balanced, meaning they have a good ratio of plant protein, complex carbohydrates, and healthy fat so you're left feeling like you had a mini-meal.

To get started, try these plant-based (and way healthier) replacements for some common snacks we all know and love:

- **Potato chips:** Choose kale chips or organic corn chips with salsa or hummus.

- **Soda pop:** Choose natural, 100 percent fruit juice, coconut water, or kombucha, which is bubbly and refreshing.

  Kombucha has become a popular fermented tea beverage you can find in health food stores, yoga studios, and craft breweries. It is said to have many detoxifying qualities, and in small doses, this elixir is full of gut-healing benefits. It aids in digestion, increases your energy, and pro-motes the growth of healthy gut flora. You can make your own kombu-cha at home (with a recipe from *Fermenting For Dummies* by yours truly [Wiley]), or you can purchase it in many flavors at health food stores.

- **Candy bars:** Make your own balanced energy bar instead (see recipe later in this chapter).

- **Fried foods:** Baked sweet-potato fries taste even better than regular fries, especially alongside a salad or some greens, or dipped in hummus.

- **Lattes or chocolate milk:** Make a chocolate smoothie for energy and natural sweetness, perfect for that midday crash.

- **Donuts:** Make a batch of muffins instead and top them with Almond Butter and Cinnamon Dip (see recipe in Chapter 15) to make your snack even more well-rounded.

Choosing Sweet or Savory Snacking

Snacks generally fall into one of two taste categories: sweet or salty (a.k.a. savory). If we don't crave one, we often crave the other — sometimes even both. But if you don't know what you're craving, I find that it works best to eat what contrasts with your last meal. That way, you can not only help balance your blood-sugar levels but also feel satisfied all day long.

Eating something savory after eating something sweet can help slow down the rate at which glucose is released into your blood, so be mindful of the last meal you ate. Did you last eat fruit salad or a smoothie containing fruit? If so, for your next meal or snack you may want to consider something savory like nuts and seeds, dried seaweed, or guacamole with corn chips. You may not realize it, but you'll feel better with this contrast.

Sometimes it's best to have both sweet and savory flavors in the same snack (slicing two carrots with one knife, so to speak). Try adding a pinch of sea salt to your apple or into your muffin batter. This little bit of salt makes the sweetness taste sweeter while helping to balance your cravings. It may sound a little strange, but it truly works. *Note:* You can technically do the reverse (add a bit of sweetener to something savory), but it doesn't often work as well.

Here are some ideas for savory munchies and add-ins:

- ✔ Non-GMO organic corn chips
- ✔ Brown rice cakes
- ✔ Gluten-free or whole-grain crackers
- ✔ Sprouted-grain tortillas
- ✔ Toasted nori or other seaweeds
- ✔ Nuts and seeds with a pinch of sea salt or splash of tamari (natural soy sauce)
- ✔ Dulse flakes

And here's a list to appeal to your sweet tooth:

- ✔ Cacao nibs or dairy-free dark chocolate chips
- ✔ Almond butter
- ✔ Apple butter
- ✔ Coconut butter or flakes
- ✔ Dried fruit, such as raisins, cranberries, goji berries, and golden berries
- ✔ Fresh fruit

Edamame Hummus

Prep time: 8 min • **Yield:** 10 servings

Ingredients	Directions
2 cups cooked, shelled organic edamame beans	*1* Combine the edamame, tahini, lemon juice, garlic, ginger, tamari, sesame oil, and olive oil in a food processor and blend until smooth.
¼ cup tahini	
¼ cup fresh-squeezed lemon juice	*2* With the motor still running, slowly add the water and sea salt until the desired consistency is reached.
2 cloves garlic, minced	
1 teaspoon chopped or minced ginger, or ½ teaspoon ground dry ginger	*3* Put the dip in a bowl and sprinkle with the black sesame seeds (if desired) and a few drops of sesame oil. Serve with brown-rice crackers.
1 teaspoon tamari	
1 teaspoon toasted sesame oil	
2 tablespoons olive oil	
¼ cup water	
½ teaspoon sea salt	
black sesame seeds (optional)	

Per serving: Calories 102 (From Fat 72); Fat 8g (Saturated 1g); Cholesterol 0mg; Sodium 141mg; Carbohydrate 5g (Dietary Fiber 1g); Protein 4g.

Sweet Pea Guacamole

Prep time: 15 min • **Yield:** 10 servings

Ingredients	Directions
1 cup frozen organic green peas, or fresh when in season, blanched	*1* Put the peas, green onions, lemon or lime juice, cumin, coriander, garlic, parsley, jalapeño (if desired), and salt into a food processor and process until well blended and smooth.
4 green onions, cut into 2-inch slices	
3 to 5 tablespoons fresh-squeezed lemon or lime juice	*2* Cut the avocados in half, remove the pits, and scoop out the flesh into a medium mixing bowl.
1 teaspoon ground cumin	
½ teaspoon ground coriander	*3* Mash the avocados and mix in the ingredients from the food processor.
¼ teaspoon powdered garlic, or 1 clove fresh garlic, peeled	
8 sprigs parsley	*4* Stir in the tomatoes and adjust the seasoning to taste.
1 jalapeño chile pepper, finely chopped, or ¼ teaspoon hot sauce (optional)	*5* Serve with organic corn tortilla chips, slices of jicama, or whole-grain crackers.
¼ teaspoon sea salt	
2 large ripe avocados	
¾ cup chopped tomatoes	

Per serving: *Calories 66 (From Fat 36); Fat 4g (Saturated 0.5g); Cholesterol 0mg; Sodium 68mg; Carbohydrate 7g (Dietary Fiber 3g); Protein 2g.*

Tip: For a flavor boost, top this dip off with an extra squirt of lime juice and a dash of sea salt.

Note: Figure 14-1 shows how to cut an avocado, remove the pit, and scoop out the meat.

Figure 14-1:
Pitting and extracting the meat from an avocado.

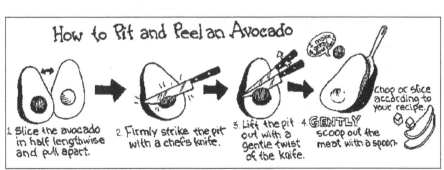

How to Pit and Peel an Avocado

1. Slice the avocado in half lengthwise and pull apart.
2. Firmly strike the pit with a chef's knife.
3. Lift the pit out with a gentle twist of the knife.
4. GENTLY scoop out the meat with a spoon.

chop or slice according to your recipe

Illustration by Elizabeth Kurtzman

Super Brazil and Goldenberry Trail Mix

Prep time: 5 min • **Yield:** 2 servings

Ingredients	Directions
1 cup brazil nuts, chopped	**1** Place all the ingredients in a large glass jar or container and shake!
1 cup unsweetened coconut flakes	
½ cup goldenberries	
¼ cup goji berries	
½ cup pumpkin seeds	
pinch of sea salt (optional)	

Per serving: Calories 1,014 (From Fat 792); Fat 88g (Saturated 37g); Cholesterol 0mg; Sodium 273mg; Carbohydrate 42g (Dietary Fiber 14g); Protein 25g.

Vary It! Swap out the brazil nuts for cashews for a decadent taste. You can also add some dairy-free dark chocolate chips or cacao nibs to get your fix of chocolate.

Note: Goldenberries and goji berries are different than your typical raisin or apricot (which can also be used). They are more tart and tangy than sweet. Both are superfood fruits with protein, antioxidants, and fiber. They can be found at health food stores.

Tip: To make this snack nut-free, choose sunflower seeds instead of brazil nuts.

Trail mix: Healthy and full of flavor

Trail mix. It's the easiest way to get a snack that's both sweet and salty. Beyond that, it's a good balance of protein, healthy fats, and carbs — even *superfoods* (foods that are densely loaded with a full spectrum of nutrients, such as vitamins, minerals, antioxidants, and protein). There's no reason, other than allergies to nuts and seeds, not to take a simple, home-made trail mix with you on the go. Keep it in your car, purse, bag, or desk. A container of trail mix is the easiest thing to make and eat.

Energizing Coconut Vanilla Chia Pudding

Prep time: 5 min, plus standing time • **Yield:** 2 servings

Ingredients	*Directions*
¼ cup chia seeds	*1* Place the chia seeds in a bowl with the hempseeds and add the coconut milk. Let the mixture stand for 5 to 10 minutes or longer so the chia seeds can gel and form a pudding.
2 tablespoons hempseeds	
½ cup coconut milk	
1 tablespoon vanilla-bean powder or vanilla extract	*2* Stir in the vanilla, goji berries or raspberries, and maple syrup.
1 tablespoon goji berries or fresh raspberries	
1 tablespoon maple syrup	*3* Let the mixture stand for another 5 minutes to soften the goji berries, then enjoy!

Per serving: Calories 319 (From Fat 198); Fat 22g (Saturated 17g); Cholesterol 0mg; Sodium 24mg; Carbohydrate 19g (Dietary Fiber 9g); Protein 9g.

Note: Chia seeds like to expand, so be sure to use a big enough bowl and enough liquid to let the chia seeds grow. You can add more coconut milk if you want a creamier consistency.

Vary It! Instead of vanilla-bean powder, try adding cocoa or cacao powder with the raspberries for a chocolate raspberry flavor.

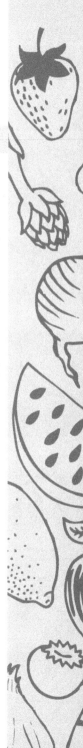

Apple Cinnamon Bites

Prep time: 10 min • **Yield:** 10–12 servings

Ingredients	Directions
½ cup chopped dates	**1** Place the dates in a food processor and blend until they form a thick paste. Place in a large bowl.
½ cup ground flaxseeds or hempseeds	
½ teaspoon ground cinnamon	**2** Stir in the flaxseeds, cinnamon, apple, oil, and apple butter, using a fork or your hands to combine. Add the oats last.
½ cup dried apple pieces, finely chopped	
2 tablespoon flax oil or coconut oil	**3** Dampen your hands with water or a touch of coconut oil and form the mixture into small balls by the spoonful.
2 tablespoons apple butter or raw honey	
⅔ cup oat flakes	**4** Put the crushed seeds on a plate or tray. Roll the date balls across the seeds, coating them well.
¼ cup crushed raw unsalted sunflower seeds, hempseeds, or pumpkin seeds	**5** Place the balls on a plate and let them set in the refrigerator for 1 hour. Store them in a glass container for a quick snack.

Per serving: Calories 143 (From Fat 63); Fat 7g (Saturated 2.5g); Cholesterol 0mg; Sodium 22mg; Carbohydrate 19g (Dietary Fiber 4g); Protein 3g.

Note: These apple-cinnamon bites keep for up to two months in the fridge or freezer. They taste extra great right out of the freezer!

Brown-Rice Krispy Bars

Prep time: 15 min • **Cook time:** 10 min, plus standing time • **Yield:** 9 servings

Ingredients	Directions
½ cup chopped almonds	**1** Preheat the oven to 200 degrees. Spread the almonds and seeds on a large baking pan and lightly toast in the oven for about 10 minutes.
¼ cup each raw, unsalted sunflower seeds, pumpkin seeds, and sesame seeds	
1 tablespoon virgin coconut oil	**2** In a large saucepan, heat the coconut oil, almond butter, and brown-rice syrup on low heat for 5 minutes. At the last moment turn off the heat, add the honey and stir over the residual heat until blended.
½ cup smooth almond butter	
½ cup brown-rice syrup	
½ cup raw honey or coconut nectar	**3** In a separate bowl, combine the rice cereal and oats and mix in the almond mixture until the grains are well coated.
2½ cups puffed-rice cereal	
1¼ cups rolled oats	**4** Add the apricots, raisins, and chocolate chips (if desired); mix well.
½ cup chopped unsulphured dried apricots	
½ cup raisins	**5** Using lightly oiled hands, press the mixture evenly into an 8-inch square cake pan greased with coconut oil. Let stand for 15 minutes in the refrigerator until firm.
¼ cup dairy-free dark chocolate chips (optional)	
	6 Cut into squares and serve.

Per serving: Calories 423 (From Fat 180); Fat 20g (Saturated 3g); Cholesterol 0mg; Sodium 21mg; Carbohydrate 56g (Dietary Fiber 6g); Protein 10g.

Vary It! For an extra boost of protein, stir 1 tablespoon of plant-based Sunwarrior protein powder (brown rice or hemp) into the almond-butter mix after removing it from the stove.

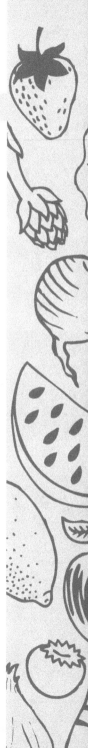

Chocolate Banana Super Smoothie

Prep time: 4 min • **Yield:** 2 servings

Ingredients	Directions
2 cups water	**1** To make a quick hemp milk base, blend the water and hempseeds in a high-speed blender until smooth.
3 tablespoons hempseeds	
2 tablespoons soaked goji berries (soak for 10 minutes)	**2** Add the remaining ingredients and blend until creamy and smooth.
1 tablespoon coconut oil or coconut butter	
1 tablespoon cacao powder	
1 tablespoon almond butter	
2 tablespoons cacao nibs	
1 to 2 scoops plant-based protein powder	
2 tablespoons chia seeds	
1 tablespoon coconut nectar	
1 cup ice	
1 banana, frozen	

Per serving: Calories 559 (From Fat 297); Fat 33g (Saturated 23g); Cholesterol 0mg; Sodium 25mg; Carbohydrate 51g (Dietary Fiber 13g); Protein 23g.

Note: You can also use the Homemade Hempseed Milk from Chapter 10 in place of Step 1, or use another type of nut or seed for variation.

Tip: Coconut oil is a great addition to this smoothie; however, it tends to clump up a bit when combined with ice. You can use coconut butter instead, which has a creamier texture (like a nut butter) with all the fiber intact. Either will work, and both taste delicious.

Cacao or cocoa

There's a difference between cacao and cocoa. Cacao is the bean from which chocolate is made. It's chocolate's rawest form and often shows up in recipes as "cacao nibs." Cocoa is created when the cacao beans are processed. Although delicious, cocoa isn't as well rounded in nutrients as cacao, which is considered by many to be a superfood.

I suggest that you use cocoa in baking and other heated desserts and cacao in raw snacks that don't require any cooking, such as Chocolate Avocado Pudding (find the recipe in Chapter 13) or a smoothie.

Zesty Kale Krisps

Prep time: 10 min • **Cook time:** 30 min to 8 hrs • **Yield:** 8 servings

Ingredients	*Directions*
1 bunch of kale, washed and torn	*1* Place the kale in a large mixing bowl by itself.
¼ cup tahini	*2* Combine the rest of the ingredients in a blender and blend until smooth to get a thick consistency. You may have to add a bit of water.
2 to 3 tablespoons tamari	
2 tablespoons apple-cider vinegar	
1 clove garlic	*3* Pour the mixture over the kale and massage thoroughly with your hands to coat the kale. Make sure the mixture covers the kale well.
juice of half a lemon	
¼ teaspoon sea salt	*4* Cook the kale chips in either a dehydrator or an oven:
2 tablespoons nutritional yeast	**In the dehydrator:** Place the kale onto two dehydrator trays and dehydrate for 4 to 8 hours at 115 degrees. Rotate the kale occasionally to dry uniformly.
	In the oven: Place the kale on parchment paper on a baking sheet and bake at 200 degrees or your oven's lowest setting for about 30 minutes. Keep an eye on them and turn them often to make sure they dry evenly.

Per serving: Calories 71 (From Fat 45); Fat 5g (Saturated 0.5g); Cholesterol 0mg; Sodium 342mg; Carbohydrate 4g (Dietary Fiber 1g); Protein 4g.

Vary It! Add more nutritional yeast to give your krisps a cheesier flavor.

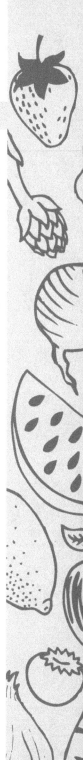

Happy Hemp Loaves

Prep time: 20 min • **Cook time:** 15–20 min • **Yield:** 6–8 servings

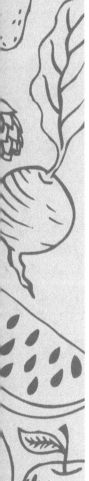

Ingredients	Directions
½ cup hemp flour	**1** Preheat the oven to 350 degrees.
1 cup brown-rice flour	
½ cup coconut flour	**2** In a large bowl, combine the hemp flour, brown-rice flour, coconut flour, baking soda, and baking powder. Set aside.
1 teaspoon baking soda	
1 teaspoon baking powder	
6 tablespoons virgin coconut oil, warmed slightly to liquefy	**3** In another bowl, combine the oil, maple syrup, applesauce, and banana and beat until well mixed.
¼ cup maple syrup	**4** Add the flax mixture and vanilla to the wet mixture and mix well.
½ cup organic applesauce or pureed apples	
1 banana, mashed	**5** Add the wet ingredients to the dry ingredients, then add the blueberries. Mix until just blended.
1 tablespoon ground flax mixed with 3 tablespoons water	**6** Pour the batter into 6 to 8 mini loaf pans greased with coconut oil so they're half full. Press the batter down to flatten. Bake for 15 to 20 minutes.
1 teaspoon vanilla	
¼ cup blueberries	**7** Remove the loaves from the oven and allow to cool on a baking rack.
pinch of sea salt	
	8 Serve with a tablespoon of almond butter or apple butter and a glass of water or almond milk for a tasty, high-protein snack.

Per serving: Calories 368 (From Fat 153); Fat 17g (Saturated 13g); Cholesterol 0mg; Sodium 379mg; Carbohydrate 50g (Dietary Fiber 11g); Protein 8g.

Note: These loafs tend to crumble a bit because they are gluten-free (the flours absorb more moisture). So be sure to press them into the loaf pans so they don't crumble as much when they come out of the oven.

Vary It: Instead of blueberries, try mixing in raisins or dairy-free chocolate chips.

Note: The high fiber content is why you should serve these with something to drink. They need some liquid to move through your body.

Chapter 15

Sauces, Sides, Dips, and Dressings

····································

In This Chapter

▶ Understanding the differences between store-bought and homemade sauces

▶ Making a meal out of sides

▶ Enhancing your meal with sides and sauces

····································

*J*azzing up your meals comes down to sauces, sides, dips, and dressings. These take your meal to the next level and give much-needed companionship to the entree on your plate. In this chapter, I give you some ideas to help you think outside your typical meal by rounding it out with these delicious extras.

Seeing the Benefits of Whipping Up Your Own Sauces, Dips, and Dressings

We all like things saucy. Sauces, dips, and dressings add texture and creaminess and can make whatever it is you sauced or dipped into taste that much better. The creamy addition of a homemade sauce, dressing, or dip can be the missing link between your wrap, quinoa, or veggie burger and ultimate deliciousness. The right topping can make the boring brilliant. It can make the same old, same old sensational. You get the idea. But beware: It only works if you make them yourself.

Store-bought or prepackaged sauces and dips are laced with extra calories, sugar, fats, and other random ingredients like corn oil, maltodextrin (a processed sugar derived from corn), and potato starches. Plus, they don't have the unique touch that you can only add at home.

Other benefits include the following:

- **Cost:** You can make your own sauces and dips from ingredients you already have at home.

- **Portion control:** Especially for couples and individuals, sometimes a prepackaged sauce or dip is just too much to use. When you make your own, you determine the amount.

- **Variety:** You don't get stuck working your way through that giant jar of marinara sauce until it's gone. When you make your own sauce, you can easily try different flavors — even during the same meal.

If you're taking all this time to make the rest of your meal healthy and delicious, why ruin it with a toxic store-bought sauce? Make sure that all the ingredients in your gorgeous veggie-based dishes are complementary and enhance the flavors of the main event.

Here are the basic components of sauces, dips, and dressings:

- **Base:** Whether it's oil, nut butter, bean, tomato sauce, or fruit juice, the base of your dressing, dip, or sauce should be thick and rich to lend itself as the carrier for the other ingredients.

- **Vinegar or acid:** Whether it's apple-cider vinegar, lemon juice, or balsamic vinegar, most dressings require an acid (although not all sauces do).

- **Oil:** Using a cold-pressed or pure oil can be an amazing addition to your sauce, dressing, or dip. It adds the richness needed to round out the flavors. The best oil to use is olive oil. It lends good flavor and has wonderful health benefits.

- **Thickener:** Try using Dijon mustard, tahini, miso, or seeds to thicken up your sauces, dips, and dressings. These also help bind the ingredients together, keeping everything smooth and creamy.

- **Added flavors:** These can come in the form of spices, herbs, or even sweeteners, such as maple syrup or honey. This is what takes your dressing, dip, or sauce over the edge, making it unique and distinguished.

Adding Variety with Sumptuous Sides

It's all about the sides. If you have nothing to put on your plate beside your main course, the plate looks very empty. It's your sides that make a meal whole. They're also the perfect platform to make your meal special.

Whether your side is greens and mushrooms or roasted potatoes, make sure you have enough variety, color, texture, and balance to make your lunch or dinner that much more exciting. Of course, nothing is wrong with pairing up your sides with some of the snack options I mention in Chapter 14 (tapas, anyone?).

Consider this: If your entree remains the same for a few meals, but you change up your sides, it'll still feel like you're eating from different menus. It's a perfect approach for those hectic weekday dinners.

These ideas for sides will get your creative wheels turning:

- ✔ Sautéed leafy, green veggies, such as spinach, kale, collards, or chard, with a small amount of olive oil and garlic

- ✔ Steamed broccoli, asparagus, and green beans topped with Tahini-Miso Gravy

- ✔ Baked sweet potato, roasted squash, or spaghetti squash

- ✔ Cooked whole-grain noodles or grains served with one of the sauce recipes in this chapter

To keep meals hearty and interesting, opt for two different kinds of veggies — one green and one root (for example, sautéed greens and yam fries) — or try serving several sides to make a complete meal.

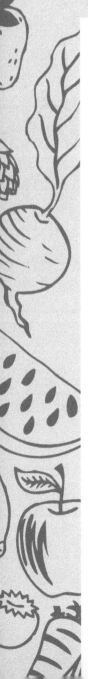

Garlic Oregano Yam Fries

Prep time: 15 min • **Cook time:** 35–45 min • **Yield:** 4 servings

Ingredients	Directions
6 to 8 medium yams or sweet potatoes	**1** Preheat the oven to 300 degrees.
2 cloves garlic, minced	**2** Cut the yams into wedges or chunks and set aside. In a bowl, combine the garlic, pumpkin seeds, oregano, basil, coconut oil, and sea salt.
2 tablespoons coarsely chopped pumpkin seeds	
1 tablespoon oregano	**3** Add the yams, stirring with your hands to make sure all of the pieces are covered with the mixture.
1½ tablespoons basil	
2 to 4 tablespoons coconut oil	**4** Spread the yams on a baking tray lightly oiled with coconut oil. Bake for about 45 minutes, or, if you prefer them crispier, leave them in the oven for an extra 10 to 20 minutes.
sea salt to taste	

Per serving: Calories 254 (From Fat 81); Fat 9g (Saturated 6g); Cholesterol 0mg; Sodium 235mg; Carbohydrate 40g (Dietary Fiber 6g); Protein 4.5g.

Rosemary Cauliflower Mashed Potatoes

Prep time: 5 min • **Cook time:** 45 min, plus standing time • **Yield:** 8 servings

Ingredients	Directions
3 cups water	**1** Bring the water to a boil in a large pot.
1 cup millet, rinsed	
1 head cauliflower, chopped into florets	**2** Place the rinsed millet in the boiling water, reduce the heat to low, and simmer for 25 minutes.
1 clove garlic	**3** Add the cauliflower and garlic and continue to simmer for another 20 minutes.
2 tablespoons olive oil	
¼ cup chopped fresh rosemary	**4** Test the cauliflower with a fork to make sure it is soft. Turn off the heat and let it stand for another 10 minutes.
½ teaspoon sea salt	
	5 Using a potato masher, mash the cauliflower until you get a thick, creamy texture.
	6 Stir in the olive oil, rosemary, and sea salt.

Per serving: Calories 133 (From Fat 45); Fat 5g (Saturated 0.5g); Cholesterol 0mg; Sodium 139mg; Carbohydrate 20g (Dietary Fiber 2.5g); Protein 3g.

Note: Serve this dish with Tahini-Miso Gravy for a perfect side dish to a hearty plant-based meal.

Vary It! Try using turnips, parsnips, squash, carrots, or beets instead of cauliflower for a different color and flavor.

Tip: For a really creamy texture with a unique flavor, try roasting the cauliflower and garlic in an oven at 300 degrees for 30 minutes instead of simmering it. Then combine the cauliflower, garlic, and cooked millet and mash them together.

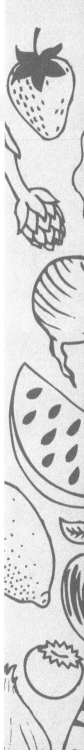

Spinach Almond Patties

Prep time: 20 min • **Cook time:** 30 min • **Yield:** 10 servings

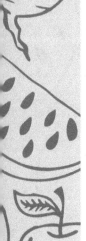

Ingredients	*Directions*
4 cups fresh spinach, washed, dried, and stems removed	*1* Preheat the oven to 350 degrees.
1 medium onion, chopped	*2* Place the spinach and onion in a food processor and blend on high until they are wet and blended. Add the bread crumbs, ¾ cups almonds, olive oil, tamari, rice flour, and dill and blend until all the ingredients are combined to form a paste.
1¼ cups wheat-free bread crumbs	
1½ cups ground almonds, or ground almond meal, divided	
2 tablespoons olive oil	*3* Fill a small bowl with water for wetting your hands while flattening the mixture into patties. Place the remaining ¾ cup ground almonds on a large plate.
2 tablespoons tamari	
½ cup brown-rice flour	
1 teaspoon dried dill	*4* Flatten the spinach mixture into 10 to 12 patties about 2 inches wide and 1 inch thick. Press them into the ground almonds, coating the outside of each patty.
	5 Place the finished patties on a lightly oiled cookie sheet. Cook for 30 minutes.
	6 Allow the patties to cool on the cookie sheet and then place them in a bowl or on a platter.
	7 Serve the patties in wraps or on sprouted-grain buns, along with a fresh salad, steamed greens, brown rice, or quinoa.

Per serving: Calories 214 (From Fat 117); Fat 13g (Saturated 1g); Cholesterol 0mg; Sodium 317mg; Carbohydrate 21g (Dietary Fiber 5 g); Protein 5g.

Note: These patties should be approximately the size of a small burger or slider.

Vary It! Instead of making flat patties, you can roll the mixture into balls about the size of a ping-pong ball.

Collards with Portobello Mushrooms

Prep time: 5 min • **Cook time:** 20–25 min • **Yield:** 10 servings

Ingredients	Directions
¾ **pound collard greens**	**1** Wash the collards, remove the stalks, and stack 4 to 5 leaves. Roll the leaves like a cigar and slice into thin ribbons.
1 cup water	
2 tablespoons olive oil	**2** To steam the collards, place the water in the bottom of a pot with a lid and bring the water to a boil. Add the collards to a steaming basket and place the basket in the pot.
2 teaspoons minced garlic	
⅓ **cup thinly sliced scallions**	
2 to 3 portobello mushrooms, cut into thin slices	**3** Cover and steam over medium heat for 5 minutes, stirring occasionally. Remove the collards from the pot and set aside.
salt to taste	
	4 Heat the oil in a skillet over medium heat. Add the garlic and scallions and sauté for 30 seconds to 1 minute. Turn the heat to medium high and add the mushrooms and a pinch of salt to draw out some liquid. Cook for 5 to 6 minutes, stirring constantly, until the mushrooms are tender.
	5 Reduce the heat to low, stir in the cooked collards, cover, and cook for another 5 minutes until warm.

Per serving: Calories 39 (From Fat 27); Fat 3g (Saturated 0g); Cholesterol 0mg; Sodium 161mg; Carbohydrate 2g (Dietary Fiber 1 g); Protein 1g.

Note: Collards are one of the toughest greens to break down, so they require a bit of steaming at the beginning to start the cooking process. However, you can skip Steps 2 and 3 and simply sauté the collards in the pan with the mushrooms, but the cooking time will be closer to 10 minutes.

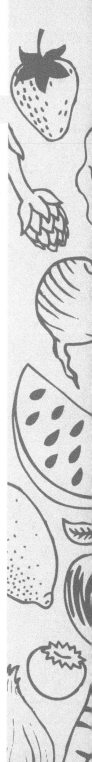

White Bean Dip with Dill

Prep time: 5 min • **Cook time:** 45 min • **Yield:** 8–10 servings

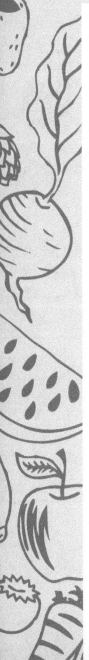

Ingredients	*Directions*
Two 14-ounce cans navy beans, rinsed and drained, or 1 cup dry beans, soaked overnight	**1** In a large pot, cook the beans and kombu in 4 cups of water for 45 to 60 minutes.
½-inch piece of kombu	**2** Put the garlic, lemon juice, and half of the beans into a blender or food processor and blend well.
2 cloves garlic	
¼ cup fresh-squeezed lemon juice	**3** Add the remaining beans, tahini, olive oil, salt, and pepper and blend until smooth. (Add water if a thinner consistency is desired.)
2 to 4 tablespoons tahini	
1 tablespoon olive oil	**4** Transfer the spread to a bowl and stir in the dill.
salt and pepper to taste	
1 bunch fresh dill or basil, finely chopped	**5** Serve with a side of whole-grain or gluten-free crackers and veggies, or scoop 2 tablespoons of dip onto a wrap or sprouted-grain bread for a sandwich.

Per serving: Calories 125 (From Fat 36); Fat 4g (Saturated 0.5g); Cholesterol 0mg; Sodium 70mg; Carbohydrate 17g (Dietary Fiber 7g); Protein 6g.

Vary It! Try this same dip with different beans such as chickpeas, black beans, kidney beans, or lentils.

Tip: If you want the beans to be nice and soft for pureeing, cook them for at least 60 minutes. You can also cook them overnight in a slow cooker on low.

Almond Butter and Cinnamon Dip

Prep time: 3 min • **Yield:** 2 servings

Ingredients	*Directions*
¼ cup almond butter	*1* Place all the ingredients in a bowl and stir with a fork or spoon to combine.
1 teaspoon cinnamon	
1 tablespoon raw honey or maple syrup	*2* Enjoy this dip with sliced apples, bananas, or pears for a nourishing and balanced snack. It can also be spread onto whole-grain toast, crackers, or rice cakes.

Per serving: Calories 231 (From Fat 162); Fat 18g (Saturated 2g); Cholesterol 0mg; Sodium 73mg; Carbohydrate 16g (Dietary Fiber 4g); Protein 7g.

Tip: This is a great dip to eat as an energizing snack before a workout.

Vary It! If you are allergic to nuts, use sunflower seed butter, tahini, or hempseed butter as an alternative and it will taste just as delicious.

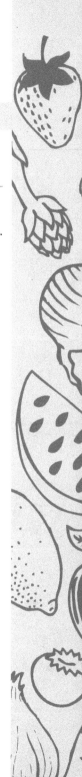

Orange Maple Marinade

Prep time: 5 min, plus standing time • **Yield:** 3–6 servings

Ingredients	Directions
¼ cup fresh orange juice	*1* Mix all the ingredients in a small glass bowl and stir with a fork or a spoon.
2 tablespoons tamari	
2 tablespoons grapeseed oil or olive oil	*2* Let it sit for at least 10 minutes to absorb the flavors.
1 tablespoon maple syrup	*3* Serve over tofu or tempeh, which will absorb the marinade's flavor.
2 tablespoons minced onions	
1 clove of garlic, minced	

Per serving: Calories 118 (From Fat 81); Fat 9g (Saturated 0.5g); Cholesterol 0mg; Sodium 672mg; Carbohydrate 8g (Dietary Fiber 0g); Protein 2g.

Tip: Warm the marinade in the oven before serving it over tofu, tempeh, or beans. The heat brings out the flavors, making it taste even better.

Note: Mincing an onion is different from mincing garlic. An onion is bigger, which makes it easier to handle, but then you have the problem of the onion causing your eyes to tear. Sometimes you just can't win! Figure 15-1 shows how to mince an onion.

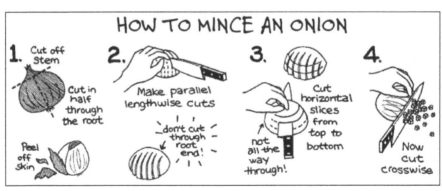

Figure 15-1: Knowing how to mince an onion comes in handy.

HOW TO MINCE AN ONION

1. Cut off stem. Cut in half through the root. Peel off skin
2. Make parallel lengthwise cuts. don't cut through root end!
3. Cut horizontal slices from top to bottom. not all the way through!
4. Now cut crosswise

Illustration by Elizabeth Kurtzman

Balsamic Maple Dressing

Prep time: 5 min • **Yield:** 4 servings

Ingredients	Directions
½ cup olive oil	**1** Place all the ingredients into a bowl, blender, or glass jar and mix until combined to form a thick dressing.
¼ cup balsamic vinegar	
1 tablespoon Dijon mustard	**2** Serve this dressing on a fresh bed of greens or on top of quinoa, farro, or brown-rice pasta.
1 clove of garlic, minced	
1 tablespoon maple syrup	
pinch of sea salt	

Per serving: Calories 267 (From Fat 243); Fat 27g (Saturated 3.5g); Cholesterol 0mg; Sodium 219mg; Carbohydrate 6g (Dietary Fiber 0g); Protein 0g.

Vary It! Swap apple-cider vinegar for the balsamic vinegar and honey for the maple syrup to make this a honey-Dijon dressing.

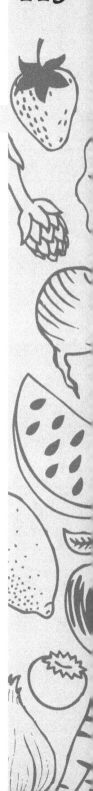

Tahini-Miso Gravy

Prep time: 5 min • **Cook time:** 5 min • **Yield:** 4 servings

Ingredients	Directions
¼ cup tahini	**1** Place all the ingredients in a small blender and blend until smooth and creamy. Or place the ingredients in a glass bowl and use a fork or whisk to combine.
2 tablespoons brown-rice miso	
1 tablespoon tamari	**2** Serve alongside steamed greens, on a fresh salad, or with any grain, such as brown rice, quinoa, or millet.
2 tablespoons brown-rice vinegar	
2 to 4 tablespoons water	

Per serving: Calories 110 (From Fat 72); Fat 8g (Saturated 1g); Cholesterol 0mg; Sodium 632mg; Carbohydrate 5g (Dietary Fiber 1g); Protein 4g.

Vary It! For a tangy variation, swap out the brown-rice vinegar for fresh orange juice or apple-cider vinegar.

Note: This sauce tastes especially good on Rosemary Cauliflower Mashed Potatoes (see the recipe earlier in this chapter).

Basil Spinach Pesto

Prep time: 10 min • **Cook time:** 5 min • **Yield:** 8 servings

Ingredients	Directions
¼ cup pine nuts or hempseeds	*1* Place all the ingredients into a food processor or blender and pulse for a few minutes until well combined. Use a spatula to scrape down the sides.
2 cups fresh basil, washed and stemmed	
1 cup fresh spinach, washed and stemmed	*2* Serve the pesto on top of brown-rice pasta, brown rice, or quinoa. You can even use it as the base for a pizza on a sprouted-grain tortilla or homemade pizza crust.
¼ cup olive oil	
1 to 2 cloves of garlic	
2 tablespoons fresh-squeezed lemon juice	
1 teaspoon white miso paste	
1 tablespoon raw honey or coconut nectar	
sea salt and pepper to taste	

Per serving: Calories 103 (From Fat 90); Fat 10g (Saturated 1g); Cholesterol 0mg; Sodium 87mg; Carbohydrate 4g (Dietary Fiber 1g); Protein 1g.

Vary It! Instead of spinach, try using kale.

Tip: If you use hempseeds, grind them separately first and then add the remaining pesto ingredients.

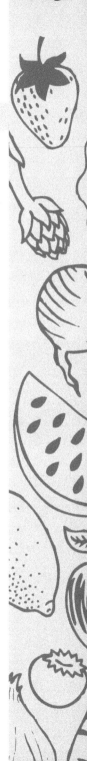

Part IV
Plant-Based for All Stages of Life

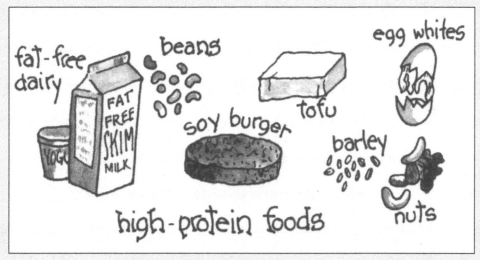

Illustration by Elizabeth Kurtzman

 Hosting a holiday or other large gathering may be a bit stressful, but it's one way to guarantee that plant-based dishes are on the menu. Head to www.dummies.com/extras/plantbaseddiet and check out the free article about planning a large meal.

In this part . . .

- ✔ Get tips for sticking to your plant-based diet when dining out and attending or hosting holiday celebrations.

- ✔ Continue to enjoy a healthy plant-based diet during pregnancy.

- ✔ Discover how to get children of any age to try (and maybe even like) plant-based foods.

- ✔ See how a plant-based diet meshes with fitness training at all levels.

- ✔ Keep up with your nutritional needs as you age.

Chapter 16

Navigating Restaurants and Special-Occasion Dining

. . . .

In This Chapter

▶ Finding veggie-friendly restaurants

▶ Navigating restaurant and takeout menus

▶ Making get-togethers extra special on a plant-based diet

▶ Sharing your plant-based lifestyle with others

. . . .

*T*here's nothing worse than getting together with your friends or family to share a meal, whether at someone's home or at a restaurant, only to find nothing you can eat. What should be a happy and enjoyable experience quickly turns into a frustrating one.

Although eating out when you're on a special diet can indeed be challenging, finding plant-based options may be easier than you think — certainly a lot easier than it was 30 years ago. More and more restaurants in more cities are able to accommodate plant-based diets. Heck, some places go beyond simply accommodating and produce some really stellar, complex dishes that are entirely plant-based. And then there are restaurants that are entirely plant-based! In a lot of ways, this is the golden age for plant-based eaters — stigma is down, availability is up.

Still, I can offer some tricks of the trade to help you leave the party with a belly full of yummy food, not one that's growling. This chapter outlines how to successfully navigate meals you eat outside of your own kitchen. It also covers what the plant-based cook can do when hosting a dinner party for non-plant-based eaters.

As someone who eats a predominantly organic and non-genetically modified diet, I sometimes have a hard time when I dine out, even though I've been doing it for a while now. All I can say is that you have to do your best and make whatever choices you can in the moment.

The Ins of Dining Out: Being a Proactive Plant-Based Eater

When eating a plant-based diet, preparing the majority of your meals yourself is typically the easiest way to make sure you get enough to eat. Not to mention, it's nice to become self-sufficient, enjoy the cooking process, and save some money, too!

Sometimes, however, dining out is on the agenda. Sometimes these meals are on your terms, and sometimes they're not. Either way, you can find ways to make sure your plant-based needs are met. In the following sections, I offer suggestions on enjoying a restaurant meal while sticking to your plant-based lifestyle.

Finding plant-friendly establishments

Good places for plant-based eaters to eat *do* exist — and you can find them. If you happen to be in a big city, it's probably easier to find amazing little cafés and restaurants that feature specialty vegetarian delights. If you live in a not-so-big city, you may have to be a little extra savvy, but it's not hard to do your research and find places to eat that suit your lifestyle (and maybe even your family members' and friends' lifestyles, too).

A restaurant doesn't have to be a hippie, veggie-loving cafe to be plant-based friendly; you can find options almost anywhere. You actually may end up frequenting mainstream restaurants because they typically have more options that can accommodate many types of diets.

Here are some good ways to discover plant-friendly restaurants that can meet your dietary needs:

✔ **Go online:** One of the best ways to find restaurants that can accommodate your needs is to run searches on the Internet before venturing out. Several websites provide resources for restaurants, markets, cafes, and other stores that are accommodating. Happycow.com is an amazing online resource that displays all the vegetarian and health-inspired eateries and stores in a city. It's searchable by region and diet (vegan, vegetarian, or veg-friendly), gives you price ranges, and includes user reviews.

✔ **Ask around at restaurants:** When you find a place, don't be shy about asking about other places to try. Not only will the restaurant owner and staff members know about similar restaurants in the area, but regular patrons will have the pulse on other good places to eat.

✔ **Pick up local newspapers and free health magazines:** Pay attention to the newspaper racks on the street and in public places. Look for a local magazine or paper that lists all the restaurants in the area; these listings are often categorized by food type, making it easier to find places that cater to plant-based eaters. You may even find some discounts!

✔ **Visit farmers' markets, trade shows, and other local fairs and festivals:** Attending local events is a great way to sample good food and get to know the owners of restaurants that serve the type of food you're looking for. Chat up your neighbors, and get to know your city in a whole different light.

✔ **Hit up social media and folks you know:** Don't forget about the old adage, "It's not what you know; it's whom you know." You may know people in your circle who are experts on veggie dining; you just may not know it yet. Do you have a co-worker who seems to eat healthfully and is into fitness? Ask him if he has any suggestions. What about fellow parents or teachers at your kids' school? And if you're on any social-media sites, make sure to ask for suggestions there.

If you have any doubts about a particular restaurant, just call ahead to ask whether it has plant-based options. Another idea is to pull up the menu online. This is especially helpful if you're dining with a group of people who have mixed eating preferences — this way, you can see whether there's something for everyone to eat.

Navigating menus

When you're in the restaurant, it's time to navigate the menu and see what's in it for you — which could take some manipulation. This may sound wrong, but it's not.

The first step is to stop seeing the menu as divided into sections. It doesn't so much matter *where* the item is listed, only that it's listed at all. As long as it's listed, you can typically order it in any format you like. Knowing how to work with what you've got is your key to dining as a plant-based king or queen.

You're the customer, and there's nothing wrong with ordering what you want in the way you want it. Although some restaurants don't accommodate special requests (there's usually a note on the menu indicating such), most restaurants will accommodate you and see to it that you feel just as important as anyone else. Sometimes the staff may even go above and beyond.

Making entrees work for you

Anything on the menu is fair game for your entree. The dishes may be listed in the entree section or as a salad, soup, or appetizer. Learn to read the menu without sections, and you won't have to despair if all the entrees contain meat.

Some entrees are easier to modify than others. You can swap out meat or fish in most stir-fries, salads, and pastas. Depending on the options the restaurant has, you can usually substitute extra veggies, beans, tofu, avocado, or even nuts. Even for steak and fish dishes, you can possibly swap for a portobello mushroom or grilled tofu. Of course, this all depends on the type of restaurant you're in and what else it has available.

Some restaurants may offer veggie burgers as an entree. However, be sure to ask what the source is, whether it is soy-based, legume-based, or made from whole grains. Also note that most veggie burgers served in restaurants are frozen and not freshly made, and some of those varieties have traces of dairy. Ask as many questions as you like so you can use your educated discretion.

Sticking with sides

I've found that at restaurants that aren't 100 percent plant-based, your best bet is sometimes going with sides — an approach I like to call "visiting the side bar." If there isn't a main dish on the menu that suits your needs, then sides may become your best friend. You can eat only so many pastas and stir-fries before you get bored with the same meals. At least you can get creative with sides.

Any of the following items may show up in the sides section of a menu, so be on alert that any combination of at least three of them can make up your dinner. (This is certainly not an exhaustive list.) Just ask for some olive oil and lemon juice or — if you're lucky — a delicious plant-based sauce that is already on the menu.

- **Veggies:** Steamed greens; side salads; steamed, grilled, or roasted veggies; shredded beets or carrots; sauerkraut, cucumber slices; and veggie sticks

- **Fruits:** Any fresh fruit

- **Cooked grains:** Brown rice, quinoa, and wild rice

- **Starches:** Baked potatoes or sweet potatoes, sweet-potato french fries (be sure to ask whether they're breaded), whole-grain or gluten-free pasta with olive oil, whole-grain bread, crackers, and wraps

- **Proteins:** Baked tofu or grilled tempeh, plain beans, baked beans or bean salads, edamame, tofu scrambles, nuts, and seeds

- **Soup:** Pureed or chunky veggie soup

- **Hummus**

Note: Many restaurants have a menu section dedicated to side dishes and building a combo plate. Be sure to look out for it on the menu!

Always be sure to ask what these side items are cooked in. Some restaurants regularly use butter, milk, or cream. You can ask for yours plain or with another option (such as olive oil, lemon, and garlic).

Asking for what you want

Sometimes you have to ask questions to figure out whether a food listed on the menu meshes with your needs. If you're assertive but polite, your server should be willing to help you put together a satisfying meal. One idea to break the ice when it's your turn to order is to announce in a jovial manner,

"I apologize in advance — I'm the difficult one!" You can also go the earnest route: "I have special dietary restrictions, but I don't want to make it hard on you — can you help me order?" Just be sure to be clear and concise, because no one likes the nitpicky person at the table.

Depending on the restaurant, you may have many or just a few options to get creative with, but either way, you're probably going to have to ask some questions. Asking the following questions is the foundation to your dining enjoyment.

Ask these questions about the ingredients:

- What kind of oils do you use?
- Is this gluten-free or wheat-free?
- Is there chicken or beef stock in this soup?
- Is there fish sauce or stock in this?
- Is there anchovy paste in this salad dressing or sauce?
- Is there dairy, cream, milk, or butter in there?
- Is there egg in that bread or pasta?
- Is there anything not on the menu that I can order?

You probably shouldn't ask all of these questions at once; use them sparingly. Remember to be assertive, not annoying.

Ask these questions about preparation and serving:

- Is a different grill/pan/pot used for tofu, tempeh, and veggies?
- Is this deep-fried in the same fryer as meat?
- Can you serve that on the side?
- Can you hold the dressing or put the dressing on the side?
- Can you steam this for me?
- Can you substitute avocado for cheese?
- Can I have gluten-free or whole-grain bread instead?
- Can you bring olive oil and balsamic vinegar on the side?
- Can I have just sides?
- Can you make my pasta without meat sauce?
- Can you make my pizza without cheese?
- Can I get steamed greens or grilled veggies instead?
- Can I get a salad instead of (potatoes, rice, pasta, meat, and so on)?
- Do you have tofu or beans to put into my stir-fry or pasta?

Eating Delivery and Takeout, Veggie Style

Depending on your lifestyle, you may often order food for delivery or take-out. However, as a plant-based eater, you may notice difficulty with ordering healthfully and in a way that provides you with a well-rounded meal. Because most take-out food is categorized by culture, I give you a little guide to the best plant-based items to order, based on cuisine. (***Note:*** Any of these suggestions is valid for dining at the restaurant, as well.)

Mediterranean

I find Mediterranean to be one of the easiest cuisines from which to order. You have so many options, especially when doing delivery or takeout, because you can supplement the meal with your own fresh salad and whole-grain or gluten-free breads or crackers for dips. Here are some good items to try:

- Lentil soup
- Hummus
- Baba ghanoush (Just make sure it's tahini based and not mayonnaise based.)
- Rice with lentils
- Grilled vegetable skewers
- Stuffed grape leaves (sometimes called *dolmas*)
- Roasted cauliflower or potatoes
- Falafel (request baked, if possible)
- Baked beans

Japanese

Japanese food tends to be pretty safe for plant-based diners; however, watch out for preservatives, MSG, and added sugars. Typically, you can eat a plant-based, gluten-free meal that is loaded with veggies. Try these:

- Miso soup (Make sure it uses vegetable stock, not fish stock.)
- Steamed edamame
- Tofu stir-fry
- Steamed greens

- Brown rice
- Brown-rice vegetarian rolls
- Seaweed salad
- Steamed tofu

Some seaweed salads are made with octopus, so be sure to ask beforehand.

Chinese

Chinese food is one of the most common forms of takeout. People just love their noodles and rice. However, be mindful of the oils and sauces, as many Chinese restaurants use poor sources of both. Feel free to ask for low sauce and oil. Most should accommodate you. Here's what I suggest the next time you order Chinese food:

- Vegetable consume
- Steamed greens
- Steamed tofu
- Green vegetables and mushrooms
- Sautéed eggplant
- Stir-fried green beans
- Steamed brown rice
- Vegetable chow mein

Italian

Italian food can be limited in terms of plant-based options, but you can usually find something. More and more, Italian restaurants have gluten-free and/ or whole-grain options for pizzas and pastas, so be sure to ask or look for the fine print, asterisks, and parentheses on the menu. Look for these options:

- Garden salad or other green salad with vinaigrette
- Whole-grain or gluten-free pasta with tomato sauce, olive oil and garlic, or vegan pesto sauce
- Whole-grain or gluten-free pizza with veggies

Be sure to ask whether the pasta noodles are made with eggs.

Thai

Just as with Japanese cuisine, you can usually find lots of plant-based options on a Thai menu. However, many Thai restaurants offer white noodles and rice as a default, so always ask for brown rice. Also ask about sauces that are oily, are fish- or oyster-based, or have added sugars and preservatives. Otherwise, here are some good choices:

- Raw rice-paper rolls with fresh veggies (Be sure not to order the fried version. Often the ones you want are called *spring rolls*, and the fried ones are called *egg rolls*. But sometimes spring rolls are fried, too, so be sure to ask.)
- Mango salad
- Green salad
- Vegetable curry
- Vegetable pad Thai with tofu or extra veggies (Read carefully or ask about this, as many places serve the dish with egg or meat as a default.)
- Brown rice
- Steamed greens or other vegetable stir-fries
- Marinated eggplant

Mexican

Mexican restaurants are definitely popular. People love their guacamole! Watch out for meat, cheese, and sour cream. You may also want to ask whether the refried beans are made with lard. Other than that, you should be safe with beans, rice, and tortillas. Luckily you can choose some of these plant-based options:

- Guacamole or salsa with corn chips
- Black-bean soup
- Vegetable burrito, taco, or quesadilla (no cheese or sour cream)
- Tortilla salad with beans and rice
- Veggie nachos (no cheese or sour cream)

Celebrating Holidays and Special Occasions

When it comes to holidays and parties, you may think you have to give in and go with the flow. You may think it's too much effort or not worth it to stay on your plant-based diet, as no one wants to eat what you're eating, or maybe you just want an excuse to "indulge" and cheat a little. But stay true to yourself — not only is this the perfect time to impress friends and family with your new skills, interest, and lifestyle, but you can also experiment with new recipes that may be different from everyone's day-to-day cuisine.

This isn't a time to fall off track! Stay motivated to stick to the choice you made to be a plant-based eater and now a plant-based partier. The following sections explain how to do just that, whether you're attending an event hosted by someone else or throwing your own get-together.

Being a gracious guest

The best way to be a great guest is to bring something. I never attend a party or dinner without bringing a dish. Not only do I cover my own needs by making sure I have something to eat, but I'm also a great guest because I share. I do this even when I'm not asked because it's just easier that way.

I usually bring at least two to three items. That way, I'm at least covered for a full meal (not just salad). Plus, I seem super generous, too!

Please be mindful that this suggestion is best for informal gatherings and potluck-style parties and may not be a good idea for formal dinner parties unless you communicate your intentions with the host. The last thing you want to do is offend someone who has spent a great deal of time putting together an amazing meal. At the very least, make sure the hosts know your restrictions; maybe they have a perfect meal already planned for you. You can ask beforehand so you're not surprised by anything.

At the very least, plan ahead and maybe eat a little something before you go to a party. Or bring a small snack that no one will notice if you step out for a few moments to eat it. The bottom line is that you need to feed yourself good plant-based food.

So, what dishes work best for parties and dinners? Here are some of my favorites:

- ✔ **Guacamole or bean dip:** This is a hearty dish that is simple to make and bring to any dinner or party. You can bring a variety of crackers or flatbreads, along with cut-up veggies, for dipping. Add fun, unique ingredients to your dips or garnish them with herbs and spices to make them look fancy. (See Chapter 14 for great guacamole and hummus recipes.)

- ✔ **Vegetarian nori rolls:** Use brown rice and pack these full of veggies. This is a great, easy-to-make appetizer for any party. Most people like sushi, so they'll be more willing to try (and like) a new plant-based food. (Check Chapter 11 for the recipe.)

- ✔ **Quinoa salad:** Find out what ingredients the partygoers like in dishes like rice and couscous, and just load up your quinoa with those items. That way, you're keeping it familiar while introducing a new recipe. (Chapter 11 has a great recipe to get you started.)

- ✔ **Green salad:** Don't just make a boring green salad — load it up with nuts, seeds, dried fruits, colorful vegetables, and avocado and make an interesting dressing that takes your salad to a whole new level. Or, make the kale slaw salad in Chapter 11; this is always a party pleaser!

Being a hostess with the mostess

Okay, so you're having people over for dinner — people who eat all sorts of things, including meat. Don't panic. This is your time to shine! You can make a balanced plant-based meal that everyone will love, from appetizers to desserts. But how?

First off, it's a good idea to know your crowd — meaning you want to make things they're going to like (or alternatives to their preferred dishes). Whether it's a hearty "meaty" meal of tempeh burgers, something with Asian flair like stir-fry, or something light and refreshing, be sure to try to accommodate your guests.

Second, decide whether you're going to let people know ahead of time that you're serving a plant-based meal. It depends on how you want to handle it. You can be upfront with folks so they can prepare and decide ahead of time if they want to come. Or you can let them come none the wiser and chow down on all of your delights; as they're enjoying the meal, you can make the big reveal. Or, of course, you can just make it a non-issue, no different than any other dinner. This approach is a well-meaning but sneaky trick you can use on skeptics of a plant-based diet — but you have to choose guests wisely so nobody gets mad for real. If you think you need some backup, invite a plant-based friend or supporter who'll be on your side for moral support.

If you're putting the whole meal together yourself, you may want to choose a simple menu that you can execute alone. If you're new to plant-based cooking, select either easy recipes or ones you've made before. That way, you take out the stress of trying something new. If you want a bit of help, enlist a willing friend or family member. Even if she's never cooked plant-based foods, as long as she can follow directions, she can be of service.

Here's a sample dinner-party menu that is simple to make, with enough variety and balance that you're sure to please many palates. (Just keep allergies in mind!)

- **Citrus Wild Rice and Broccoli** (see Chapter 11)
- **Black Bean Cumin Burgers** (see Chapter 12)
- **Sweet Pea Guacamole** (see Chapter 14)
- **Fresh fruit with cashew cream or Apricot Fig Oat Bars** (see Chapter 13)

Make your dessert ahead of time if it requires baking or freezing. Not only will you have a chance to re-make it if something goes wrong, but it also saves you time the night of your dinner, makes the dessert easier to cut, and even gives you time to decorate it.

If you're not up for doing the whole thing yourself (or you just want to try something different), try these unique takes on the typical dinner party:

- **Host a potluck.** This is the best way to take the pressure off of yourself and have everyone contribute to the meal. However, you must direct your guests well; otherwise, you leave some dishes open to chance and may have non-plant-based ingredients lurking in your home without knowing it. One idea is to design a menu and give everyone a recipe to make. That way, you know exactly what's coming. Or, if you don't want to seem like a control freak, just give gentle guidelines about what to bring. The last option is to be even more flexible: Make a few plant-based dishes that you can eat and have other people bring the rest of the food.

- **Offer a cooking class.** This is a fun and creative way to get your guests involved in the creation of the meal in real time. Of course, this only works if your guests are willing to take this on, or if you're willing to take a chance and surprise them. You can buy all the ingredients ahead of time, get everything organized, and set up stations, and then when people come, have them pair or group up at a station to make part of the meal. This can be a fun way to engage and socialize with one another before you eat, and the meal is that much more meaningful because everyone becomes part of the experience. I promise, the food tastes that much better to all your guests because they're involved.

Showing People Just How Fun Veggie Dining Can Be

If you choose to, you can make it your mission to inspire people to learn about plant-based diets and eat the way you do. Here are some ways to do it:

- ✔ **Take interested parties to a delicious plant-based restaurant** that serves a hearty (and maybe even upscale) meal that will impress them.

- ✔ **Impress people by sharing something homemade with them** that's really exciting and yummy, such as Chocolate Avocado Pudding (see Chapter 13).

- ✔ **Share inspiring stories of some of the health benefits** you've noticed from being on a plant-based diet.

- ✔ **Talk about some of the new foods or recipes you've discovered.** Offer to share recipes when people express an interest.

- ✔ **Invite meat-eating folks to come over for a night of taste testing.** Make your best meatlike and dairylike dishes and dare people to notice the difference! Make the meal even more interesting by letting your guests bring the meat equivalents, and then do a head-to-head blind tasting. (Remember, this is for the meat-eating folks only!)

- ✔ **Buy anyone who shows resistance a copy of your fave plant-based book (this one!).** Or, if you want to go the more economical route, e-mail links to particularly poignant articles, videos, and the like.

And, of course, here are some things *not* to do:

- ✔ **Don't make fun of or judge anyone else's food in any way.** You may feel all high and mighty in the moment, but you never want to judge what anyone else is eating. You don't want to be *that* person. Obviously, just think about how you'd feel if someone did that to you.

- ✔ **Don't talk about how much better your food is.** You don't want to be a plant-based food elitist. You likely know when you have a more delicious and healthful plate of food in front of you than someone else does. But just silently acknowledge it and don't brag about it. No one will be interested in the way you eat if you do that!

- ✔ **Don't preach; instead, lead by example.** To be honest, the less you say, the more people are drawn to you and want to know or ask more.

- ✔ **Don't get discouraged.** It may take a couple of occasions or even years for friends and family to fully get it. In fact, they may never get it, and you just have to accept that. But I promise that some will come around and not only want to try what you've made but also ask you all kinds of health questions. Sometimes plant-based eaters become the health gurus of the family, and people start to confess their ailments and ask for advice.

Chapter 17

Eating Plant-Based When You're Pregnant

*B*eing pregnant can be a wonderful, almost magical time for many women and families. It's full of excitement and anticipation. Preparations for the new arrival commence, loved ones scurry about to help, and everyone is focused on the new life that is forming. But pregnancy can also be nerve-racking. And stressful. And confusing.

With varying advice and professional guidance, it can be pretty difficult to figure out what you should do to best care for yourself and your baby. You may even begin to doubt your choice to eat a plant-based diet. But don't worry. That's why I'm here. Pregnancy is a time to make sure your plant-based nutrition is well balanced. In this chapter, I discuss concerns and how-to advice for women who are expecting. You can have your plants — and your baby, too!

Maintaining a Balanced Diet for Two

Being plant-based while pregnant is a frequent topic of concern. People often wonder whether a plant-based diet is safe for both the mother and her baby. Fortunately, I have good news — a plant-based diet is perfectly safe and may be the healthiest way to eat during pregnancy. You just have to plan carefully. Of course, you should consult your doctor, naturopath, or nutritionist if you have any concerns.

Before your pregnancy, you may want to prepare your body. If you're working toward getting pregnant within a certain time period, look at the calendar and flip back at least six months — if not a year — so you can work on getting your body in an optimal state before you have a little one on board. The more prepared and pre-loaded with good nutrients your body is, the more likely you'll conceive easily *and* go on to have an easier and more pleasant pregnancy. Now, obviously, not all pregnancies are thought out and planned that far in advance (all the more reason to stick to your plant-based diet year-round; you never know when you'll really need to benefit from it), but if you can do a bit of preparation, you'll be better off when you do get pregnant.

The first step is to change any lifestyle habits that may pose risks to your health or your baby's health. Quitting smoking and eliminating alcohol and caffeine from your diet are likely the first changes you should make. From there, you want to learn about the nutrients your body needs during pregnancy, such as protein, iron, folate, and calcium, and start building up those reserves.

The best foods for a plant-based pregnancy

Whether you need to give yourself a nutrition makeover or are already health savvy, your body is now the vessel for another life. This means that you have to work toward making your body and your baby as healthy as possible.

It's essential to understand which nutrients to incorporate during this crucial phase of life and to find out which foods contain those nutrients. The bottom line is that your body needs more calories, protein, iron, calcium, and folic acid, along with vitamins and minerals — all of which can be naturally derived from a plant-based diet. As a pregnant, plant-based woman, all you need to do is consume more of everything (well, the good things, anyway).

Note: Don't use your pregnancy as an excuse to eat more and eat the wrong kinds of foods. Use the guidelines in this section to help you plan how much to eat of each nutrient.

Try these key nutrient and food sources for a healthy plant-based pregnancy:

- ✔ **Protein:** You need to increase your protein intake during pregnancy. Ideally, you should consume approximately 50 percent more protein a day (versus when not pregnant). This is crucial for the growth and development of the baby, and it keeps you satisfied, as well. You can choose from a variety of incredible plant-based protein sources, such as beans, legumes, nuts, seeds, sprouted grains, tempeh, dark leafy greens, and sea vegetables. These foods also contain iron.

Note: Recommended protein intake is based on 0.4 grams of protein per pound of ideal body weight. You can work with these numbers to figure out how much you need. Remember, this is just a guideline.

✔ **Iron:** Getting enough iron is important to ensure a healthy rate of development for your baby and to ensure a strong and energized pregnancy for you. Your body is now making extra blood for the babe, so you need more iron than ever — about 49 milligrams a day. Focusing on iron-rich foods, such as dark beans and leafy green veggies — helps with blood-cell production.

✔ **Calcium:** This is the most essential mineral for the health of a pregnant woman, as it helps to form the bones, teeth, and muscles of your growing baby. The current recommendation is 1,000 milligrams per day. Calcium-rich sources of plant-based food include green leafy vegetables, sea vegetables, whole grains (such as quinoa and millet), nuts (such as almonds), seeds (such as hempseeds), and legumes (such as lentils and organic soy).

Calcium doesn't work alone; it needs vitamin D for proper absorption, so it's important for pregnant women to get adequate sunlight (about 15 to 30 minutes a day). Sunlight helps your body convert UVB rays into vitamin D, which then helps you absorb your calcium.

✔ **Folate and folic acid:** Folate is a B vitamin that is crucial for forming red blood cells and that aids in the growth and reproduction of other cells. It's also particularly crucial for the development of the baby's nervous system. Folate also stimulates your appetite, which helps you maintain your overall nutrient intake. You should aim to take no more than 1,000 micrograms per day. Food sources include green leafy vegetables, whole grains, beans, avocados, oranges, and bananas. If you find that you aren't getting enough folate naturally (most people on a plant-based diet don't), consider taking supplements. The synthetic, supplemental form of folate is folic acid.

✔ **Vitamin B12:** This vitamin helps you maintain a healthy nervous system and creates enough blood for you and your baby. Nutritional yeast and seaweed are good plant-based sources of B12. Sources such as tempeh and miso are also great because they're fermented, which means your body absorbs them more easily. However, you'll probably need to take a B12 supplement.

Foods to avoid during pregnancy

Because this is a plant-based book, you likely expect me to recommend avoiding animal-based products during pregnancy. Although this goes against most traditional guidelines, eating animals is harmful not only to your health but also to the environment (more on that in Chapter 25).

Because this is the most precious and vital time to nourish your growing baby, make sure that you don't compromise its development by putting certain foods or toxins in your body. I bet you know a lot of this already; however, it doesn't hurt to go over it just to make sure. While pregnant, be sure to limit or avoid:

- **Animal products:** Although meat, poultry, dairy, and fish are often recommended during pregnancy, in many cases they're harmful because the fatty tissues of animals store toxins. This can be dangerous to the fetus. Also, dairy products and eggs harbor bacteria that can be detrimental to pregnancy. The same goes for fish and shellfish, primarily because they may contain heavy metals.

- **Refined carbohydrates and sugars:** These provide very little nutritional value and add no significant value to the health of a pregnant woman. They can cause discomfort in terms of bloating and headaches.

- **Salt:** Standard iodized table salt and even kosher salt are the worst offenders, as they increases blood pressure and produce excess swelling in the body. It's doubtful you want extra fluids around your body when you're pregnant!

- **Highly processed vegetable fats:** As always, hydrogenated and trans fats are a big no-no, especially during pregnancy. A growing baby needs essential fats for proper growth, development, and brain function. See Chapter 3 for more info.

- **Alcohol:** Avoid alcohol, especially in the second and third trimesters. This can negatively affect the growth and development of your baby.

- **Caffeine:** Caffeine can interfere with the absorption of iron from vegetables and other foods. Caffeine has also been associated with low birth weight.

- **Sugar substitutes:** Chemicals like aspartame and saccharin are toxins that don't metabolize in anyone's body, especially in one that is pregnant. Chapter 3 has the rundown on these substitutes and their dangers.

- **Artificial flavors, food dyes, and nitrites:** These non-foods, often found in packaged products, don't provide your body with nourishment and can harm your and your baby's health. Flip to Chapter 8 for more on additives and packaged foods.

Some preliminary data indicates that flaxseeds should not be consumed during the last two trimesters of pregnancy, as they may cause pre-term delivery.

Talking to Loved Ones about Your Dietary Choices

You can almost count on the people in your life (other than maybe your partner) barraging you with questions about how your diet is going to impact the baby — heck, maybe they already are! From their perspective, they're just expressing their loving concerns about the dietary choices you're making. From your perspective, these conversations can be frustrating and annoying.

Before you even *get* to that point, prepare yourself (and them) with the right information. Your loved ones likely just want to know that you're okay and well taken care of. In the following sections, I offer some pointers about preparing for and having this conversation.

Getting started

Before you share your plans with and educate your loved ones, you have to fortify yourself. Now, I'm not exactly implying that this is a battle, but let's be honest — people can get pretty passionate when it comes to pregnancy. A lot of folks have ideas, opinions, and beliefs about right and wrong ways to conduct yourself during pregnancy. So before you even try to have conversations about your plant-based diet, complete these steps to make it easier:

- ✔ **Familiarize yourself with standard nutritional recommendations for pregnancy (such as the ones in this book and beyond).** You can only educate your loved ones if you're educated yourself, so make sure your nutritional knowledge is up to snuff.

- ✔ **Know what foods are going to nourish you for the course of the pregnancy.** Beyond reading this book, ask questions of your health-care provider to make sure you understand and feel comfortable with your diet — especially questions about protein, iron, and general nutrition.

- ✔ **Make sure you have a core team for ongoing questions, support, and feedback.** These allies should include a partner or friend, plus a doctor, midwife, or naturopath.

Educating your loved ones

If people are prying, they're probably doing so out of love and to make sure that you and your baby are healthy. That said, this is *your* body, *your* pregnancy, *your* baby, *your* diet, *your* — you get the picture. You have the right to do as you see fit, as long as it's in conjunction with health-care professionals and doesn't cause harm. You don't *have* to tell your family anything.

You don't have to explain one word to them. But should you want to, try these tips to make communicating your wishes as seamless as possible for you and your family:

- ✔ **Bring one of your core team members along for moral support.** It can help to have a friendly face in the crowd and someone to jump in and help answer questions.

- ✔ **Be loving and genuine, but direct and firm.** Explain as much or as little as you'd like and be patient with answering questions, but don't beat around the bush. Be clear and confident in your reasoning.

- ✔ **Show your loved ones books on healthy plant-based pregnancy and leave them lying around your home.** That way, when people come over, they not only see that you're doing your research but may also be curious enough to pick up the book and read a bit themselves.

- ✔ **Direct your loved ones to plant-based blogs and websites that have information on healthy outcomes for plant-based pregnancies.** At the very least, show them resources and articles on how to have a healthy plant-based or vegan pregnancy. A good resource for this is www.veganpregnancy.com.

- ✔ **Keep a detailed record or food diary to show everyone what you're eating and how healthy it is.** This can even be helpful for your health-care provider and for friends who may want to consider having a plant-based pregnancy.

Troubleshooting: Beating Nausea and Other Discomforts with Plants

With someone growing inside of you for nine months, you're bound to hit a few roadblocks along the way and not feel like your best self. Some pregnant women suffer from discomforts more than others do. Luckily, in the plant world, many foods can act as medicine and help to heal you. Supplementation may also be required, but that should be done under the supervision of a health-care provider. If you're having cravings, feeling dehydrated, or experiencing nausea, check out the following sections for plant-based remedies.

Intense cravings

Pregnant women are known to crave everything from dirt to french fries. You may develop cravings you don't expect. You may crave unusual combinations of foods or even foods that you've never eaten before. Other cravings may involve a certain texture, such as creamy, chewy, or crunchy. You may even hate certain foods you used to love.

Most of these cravings and shifts in taste are harmless and okay to indulge in (in moderation). Let your body enjoy what it's looking for — whether it's a texture, taste, or flavor. The good news is that the plant-based world is exceptionally abundant in these foods and can satisfy most cravings.

However, on a deeper level, your craving may be telling you that you require certain minerals or nutrients that you aren't getting enough of, such as calcium and protein. Also note that emotional cravings (a food craving brought on by an emotional need rather than a physical one) may be involved as well, so be sure to explore these. That way, you can decipher whether you need emotional support from other moms who have experienced what you're going through.

Even as a plant-based eater, don't be surprised if you crave meat or other high-protein animal-based foods. If you're craving animal food and dairy during your pregnancy as a plant-based eater, it may feel a bit confusing. Without putting too much thought into it and second-guessing that you're eating the right diet, just know that this typically means that you require more iron, calcium, or protein. Look at the section earlier in this chapter for some top food sources for these nutrients.

Try these plant-based sources to satisfy the most common cravings during pregnancy:

- ✔ **Cheese:** Nutritional yeast or avocado can be added to bread, crackers, or even popcorn. Sometimes a cup of miso soup or a handful of cashews can also be helpful.

- ✔ **Ice cream:** Try non-dairy coconut-based ice cream or Chocolate Avocado Pudding (see recipe in Chapter 13).

- ✔ **Chicken or beef:** Substitute marinated tofu or tempeh, cut into strips, or try grilling a portobello mushroom and eating it with some beans and legumes to get more iron.

Strange cravings are par for the pregnancy course. However, don't overlook the possibility of pica. This is a condition in which one craves strange and non-nutritive substances, such as dirt, clay, or even laundry detergent. Although it's not uncommon for pregnant women to experience pica, giving in to these cravings can be dangerous. If you experience cravings for non-food items, tell your health-care provider.

Dehydration

Making sure you're well hydrated during your pregnancy is key to staying healthy. This means sticking to lots of water, including warm or room-temperature water with ginger or lemon, and maybe even coconut water. This *doesn't* mean drinking coffee, lattes, sodas, or other sugar-laden drinks. These aren't beverages to which you want to expose yourself or your growing baby.

Not all herbal teas are safe to drink during pregnancy. Speak to your midwife or doctor to explore this further and find out which ones are safe to drink. Some teas to watch out for are peppermint, red raspberry leaf, chamomile, and nettle.

When you're dehydrated, your body loses electrolytes, the main salts — such as sodium and potassium — that the body requires to function. Sodium and potassium enable the nerves, cells, heart, and muscles to carry electrical impulses. It's vital to make sure you consume enough of these and stay hydrated during your pregnancy.

Unfortunately, many people rely on sports drinks for these electrolytes, but these drinks are little more than chemical concoctions containing food dyes and other scary ingredients that you don't ever want to put in your body — especially not during pregnancy.

Coconut water, sea vegetables, and natural sea salt are pure, plant-based sources of electrolytes that pose no risk when consumed regularly. Even just adding a squeeze of lemon to some water can work wonders for promoting hydration (because it makes tasteless water seem more exciting).

Nursing nausea (morning sickness)

In pregnancy language, we know *nursing nausea* more commonly as *morning sickness*, but because it can come at any point in the day, let's just talk about nausea. It's that icky, queasy feeling that turns your stomach and gives you a headache, the sweats, and just an all-over sense of blah. Not to mention, it often literally makes you sick.

Most of these symptoms are normal during the first trimester, but if you're not eating or have excessive vomiting, you may want to talk to your midwife or doctor. This can be dangerous, as you're likely dehydrated and not getting the nutrients your body needs for your growing baby.

Although everyone is different, these plant-based tips may help you get through these not-so-pleasant moments:

- ✔ Eat regular meals throughout the day that are balanced with greens and plant protein.
- ✔ If you're not in the mood to eat, at least have a protein shake with a scoop of rice-based protein and non-dairy milk.
- ✔ Keep a plate of plain rice crackers next to your bed and eat a few if you wake up in the middle of the night and immediately upon waking in the morning.

✔ Drink small amounts of *natural* electrolyte beverages, such as coconut water, to replenish your salts.

✔ Relieve your nausea by eating watermelon and drinking naturally sweetened ginger lemonade. Fresh mint is also known to calm an upset stomach. Ginger tea, either iced or hot, can be made by steeping freshly cut pieces of ginger in hot water.

✔ Eat mild foods that are free of excessive spices and flavoring, such as plain whole grains, tofu, avocado, and toast.

✔ Soothe minor heartburn and upset stomach by drinking one to two tablespoons of aloe juice. You can mix it into apple juice if you need to.

Other discomforts

Try these quick plant-based remedies for some other common pregnancy ailments:

✔ **Help ease constipation** with ½ cup applesauce mixed with one tablespoon ground chia seeds.

✔ **For headaches and body aches,** sip peppermint tea or add a few drops of peppermint essential oil to a bath.

✔ **To avoid fatigue,** build up your iron and protein stores with pumpkin seeds, apricots, figs, and green veggies.

Chapter 18

Raising Children on a Plant-Based Diet

. . . .

In This Chapter

▶ Seeing how starting young makes all the difference

▶ Feeding toddlers a plant-based diet

▶ Helping your teens make the best plant-based decisions in social situations

. . . .

I can't think of a better way to raise children than infusing their little bodies with the best nature has to offer. When you start feeding a plant-based diet to your young children, you train their palates, their brains, and their bodies to become accustomed to the taste, texture, and benefits of plants (in other words, you teach them lifelong healthy habits). The infusion of nutrition that plants give to a growing body is beyond any other category of food. The benefits of feeding your child plants at a young age include:

✔ It makes it more likely that your children will build strong immunity right from the beginning, which will help them build a healthy constitution for the rest of their lives.

✔ It significantly reduces their intake of saturated fats, cholesterol, preservatives, and additives.

✔ It takes away the risk of meat-borne illness.

Raising children on a plant-based diet is more doable than ever! This chapter takes you from birth through the teenage years and outlines different strategies for and benefits of feeding your kids plant-based diets.

Knowing What to Watch Out for When Raising Plant-Based Kids

In the interest of being thorough, I should address the common drawbacks or concerns about raising kids on a plant-based diet. One of the biggest concerns that parents seem to have is that their children won't get the right or enough vitamins and nutrients to grow strong and healthy. To do this successfully, you have to be on top of things and make sure your child gets a healthy variety and balance. Luckily, the plant world is loaded with vitamins and minerals (for a refresher, flip back to Chapter 3), but here are some tips to keep in mind:

- ✔ Make sure your pediatrician or naturopath knows and supports your decision so he or she can be on the lookout for any deficiencies that may pop up.

- ✔ Common deficiencies in plant-based kids are iron, zinc, and vitamin B12. One way to address this is to give them more foods that are rich in these sources. Nuts, seeds, and seaweeds are a great place to start.

- ✔ Don't overfeed your kids the bad stuff. A lot of parents worry that children aren't getting enough protein, for example, so they stuff them full of saturated fats and sugars. Be sure to look into all the healthy sources of plant-based protein from beans, seeds, plant-based protein powders, and fermented soy, all of which provide a healthy dose of protein.

Despite these concerns, making the choice to base your kids' diet around plants is one of the best decisions you can make.

Nurturing a Plant-Based Baby

None of us can grow up without being a baby first, and that's where a plant-based diet begins. Because a baby's food typically comes directly from his mother in the form of breast milk, it's up to her to make sure *her* diet is up to snuff. *Everything* that goes into her body comes out of her breast for her baby, so that's where you should start your efforts. A mom is essentially making a milkshake or smoothie out of everything she puts into her own body, so making sure the mom is eating plant-based is step one.

However, you may also need to consider using formula, and eventually you'll introduce solid foods. The following sections help you move from breast milk to plant-based solids.

Understanding why breastfeeding is essential for your baby

There is no better food for an infant than breast milk. The makeup of a mother's milk offers the perfect ratio of nutrients for her growing child, especially if she's eating a high-quality plant-based diet. No formula can replace what the body makes on its own. It's the most essential source of nutrition, so if you're able to breastfeed with ease, I would say that it's your role as a mother to provide your baby with this milk for as long as possible. The ideal standard is six months to a year. Some mothers even go as long as two years. Plant-based solid foods can be introduced during that time, but a healthy mom's breast milk should ideally be the only milk your baby gets unless you face breastfeeding challenges.

Note: Some women simply can't breastfeed for various reasons, be they health concerns, cultural expectations, job constraints, or the like. You have to consider your own individual situation when deciding whether to breastfeed (see more later in this chapter).

Although some folks contend that breast milk is still milk and isn't technically plant-based, that position is trumped when breast milk is totally natural and loaded with good nutrition that is beneficial to a growing baby.

Here's why breastfeeding is essential:

✔ **Better brain:** A child's brain grows most quickly during infancy, doubling its volume and reaching about 60 percent of its adult size by baby's first birthday, so this is a critical time of development. Children who are breastfed are known to have higher IQ scores. A key ingredient called DHA (docosahexaenoic acid), along with other fats, contributes directly to brain growth by providing the right substances for manufacturing myelin so that the brain's pathways can carry information. Breast milk is also rich in cholesterol; formula contains none. Cholesterol is used for building the brain and manufacturing hormones and vitamin D.

✔ **Good sugar:** The predominant sugar in breast milk is lactose, which breaks down into glucose and galactose. Galactose is a valuable nutrient for brain tissue development.

✔ **Smarter connections:** During rapid brain growth, neurons proliferate and connect with other neurons to make circuits throughout the brain. The more circuits and the better the quality of these circuits, the smarter the baby. Interaction with caregivers increases these connections. Breastfed babies feed more often and are held more closely, with more skin-to-skin contact, so each feeding encourages the growing brain to make the right connections, adding more circuits with the right nutrients.

✔ **Better breathing and hearing:** Breastfed babies develop larger nasal space and a larger u-shaped dental arch that does not infringe on the nasal passages above. Breastfed babies are also likely to have fewer ear infections and fewer allergies.

✔ **Intestinal health:** Breast milk is easier to digest and easier to pass in stools. Reflux occurs less often in breastfed babies because breast milk is emptied twice as quickly from the stomach and because breastfed babies tend to eat smaller meals.

✔ **Reduced risk of diabetes:** Breastfeeding, plus the delayed introduction of cow's milk, reduces the risk of type 1 diabetes.

✔ **Higher immunity:** One drop of breast milk contains around a million white blood cells. These cells (called *macrophages*) gobble up germs. Babies have a limited ability to produce antibodies to germs. Especially from six months to one year, when the placental antibodies are gone and the baby can't yet make his own antibodies, breast milk is important.

✔ **Better general health:** While babies breastfeed, they're protected from a variety of illnesses, and when they do become ill, they're less likely to become dehydrated.

Loading breast milk with nutrients

It's one thing to just eat a good, wholesome, plant-based diet for healthy breast milk, and it's another thing to kick it up a notch. Here are some helpful hints for producing healthy plant-based breast milk:

✔ Consume more of these foods to promote nutrient-rich milk: apricots, asparagus, green beans, carrots, sweet potatoes, parsley, and all leafy greens and grains.

✔ Drink plenty of pure, filtered water.

✔ Get plenty of rest (well, as much as you can with a newborn), as lack of sleep produces milk shortages.

As a mother who is keen to give her child only the best, you may want to consider brewing your own plant-based elixirs that will enhance breastfeeding. These herbs are examples of *galactagogues* — herbs that increase milk supply, improve the nutrient quality of your milk, and lift melancholy and mild depression:

✔ Alfalfa

✔ Blessed thistle

✔ Dandelion roots and leaves

- Marshmallow root
- Milky oats
- Nettle (leaves can also be eaten)
- Red raspberry leaves
- Slippery elm bark

Take these herbs in infusions or tinctures in doses of ½ to 1 ounce of dried herbs per liter of water, or 10 to 30 drops of tincture two to four times a day.

Understanding the ins and outs of formula

Although breast milk is best, mothers may not be able to breastfeed for all kinds of reasons:

- Personal discomfort with breastfeeding
- Difficulty with the baby latching onto the breast
- Difficulty producing milk
- A blocked duct in the breast
- A busy work schedule and no time to feed
- Presence of mercury or alcohol in the blood
- A medical condition requiring certain treatments or medications
- Breast surgery or reduction, which can prevent milk flow

Some natural formulas are made from organic and non-GMO ingredients; however, most formulas are made from cow dairy, which is unnatural, non-plant-based, and more difficult for a baby to digest. Additionally, most formulas are infiltrated with all kinds of sugars, syrups, oils, and other additives that are just not nutritive to your baby. They also lack antibodies to help with a baby's immune system and are expensive.

As a result, many families have turned to soy as an alternative. Although it's seemingly harmless, most soy in formulas is not organic, which means it has been genetically modified and also has been isolated into a form that is pretty much unreadable to the human body. Many babies develop allergies to soy later in life because of early exposure to an unnatural form of it. I definitely do not recommend soy-based formulas.

Homemade infant formula can be an option; however, it's important to make sure that the right ingredients go into it to ensure that it has enough fat, protein, and vitamin D, which are all essential to the baby's health. Some mostly vegan formula recipes are available online. However, note that many of them have a few non-plant-based ingredients that try to mimic the contents of breast milk. Again, this is only recommended for extreme cases and if breastfeeding is not an option for you.

You may want to have a formula recipe on hand just in case, even if you're not anticipating any problems with breastfeeding; emergencies do happen! You can find many versions online; some are vegan and some contain non-plant-based ingredients. Find one that resonates with you and run it by your health-care practitioner, just to be on the safe side.

Finally, some women consider using a breast-milk donor bank or getting it from another mom. Be careful, as you may have no knowledge about the diet or lifestyle of the donor. She may be a consumer of meat, coffee, fast food, or any number of undesirable diet choices. Not to mention, the breast milk from donor banks is pasteurized, which destroys all the enzymes.

Starting on solids

Choosing when (and with what) to put your infant on solids can be an overwhelming and sometimes stressful feat. Typically, infants start on solids somewhere in the range of six to nine months.

Be careful not to jump the gun before the baby is ready and hasn't fully developed the right enzymes to digest solid food. Feeding your child anything but breast milk in the first six months can increase the risk of infections, allergies, sudden infant death syndrome (SIDS), iron deficiency, and gastroenteritis in your baby.

In my opinion, it's best to wait as long as possible and to be extremely methodical about your approach to introducing solid foods, as some foods should be introduced earlier than others.

Reasons to wait on solids include:

- ✔ Baby's intestines are immature.
- ✔ Baby's tongue thrust reflex hasn't developed, and the swallowing mechanism is immature.
- ✔ Baby needs to be able to sit up.

The old-school schedules of feeding your child rice cereal, then vegetables and meats, then cheese, and so on aren't very useful anymore (or applicable to plant-based eaters). Instead, you can introduce them to simple, soft fruits and cooked vegetables as soon as they show an interest in solid foods — often by watching what you're eating or making chewing motions. This usually happens by the time they have their first couple of teeth, around seven months. Here's a suggested timeline:

- ✔ At seven months, start your baby on soft, nutrient-dense foods like pureed bananas, avocados, peaches, applesauce, and steamed broccoli.

- ✔ Around eight or nine months, introduce a few more foods, such as mashed sweet potatoes or rice cereal, mashed peas or green beans, or tofu (although watch for any signs of allergies or intolerance to soy).

Babies, when breastfed, don't need a lot of variety when they start eating solids. The food acts as a supplement, more for the experience and exposure to new things than for the nutrition (because most of their calories and nutrients come from the breast milk).

- ✔ Around one year, add things like non-dairy yogurt (coconut) and beans. Puffed rice, puffed millet, and gluten-free toasted-oat cereals are also great foods for older babies. Brown rice cakes, too.

Avoid feeding your child certain foods until your child is at least 12 to 18 months old:

- ✔ **Honey:** Can cause botulism.

- ✔ **Strawberries:** Allergenic.

- ✔ **Kiwi:** Allergenic.

- ✔ **Tomatoes:** Too acidic, which can cause a rash on their faces and little baby bums!

- ✔ **Citrus fruits:** A drop of lime or lemon is okay.

- ✔ **Nuts:** Allergenic, but a lot depends on your family's history.

- ✔ **Wheat (gluten):** Introduce gluten-free grains first and watch for signs of celiac disease.

Introducing solid foods can seem like a chore sometimes. Try these hints as you embark on this phase:

- ✔ Remember that it takes a baby 8 to 12 times of trying a new food before he adapts to a new flavor, so be patient and don't get too discouraged.

- ✔ Feed solid food at a time when milk supply is low.

✔ Feed one new food at a time.

✔ Skip introducing something new if baby is cranky or sick.

✔ Leave plenty of time for feeding; it's a long process.

Whipping up your own baby food

When feeding your children solid foods, you want to give them the best quality organic food. Even extremely low doses of pesticides are linked to cancer, birth defects, and more — particularly during fetal development, infancy, and childhood.

One way of introducing the foods I've listed earlier in this chapter (aside from offering them to your baby as they are) is to make your own baby food. It's actually fast and easy, and it saves money! You can choose exactly what goes into your baby and customize the food combinations to create new tastes and textures to suit your child as she grows. Just cut up a few extra veggies for baby and prepare them the same way (but without any spices) at the same time you're making your own dish.

Here's how to do it:

1. **Peel, core, and chop fruits or vegetables into smaller cubes so they steam more quickly.**

2. **Fill a saucepan with enough water to steam and not evaporate. Heat over high heat until boiling.**

3. **When the water is boiling, put the fruit or vegetable into a steamer basket and place it on top of the water. Steam on medium heat.**

   Dried fruits, such as apricots or prunes, must be boiled with enough water to cover them in the saucepan until they become soft.

4. **Steam until the fruit or vegetable is tender;** a knife should slide through them easily, and you should be able to mash them without resistance (denser vegetables will take longer).

5. **Empty the contents into a bowl and mash by hand, in a blender, or in a food processor before adding any water.**

6. **Add water by very small amounts until you get the consistency you want.**

   Add a little breast milk to the puree for palatability and ease of digestion because of the rich source of probiotics.

7. **Puree until it's the texture of smooth, thick soup;** as baby gets older, reduce the water and leave a few lumps in the food.

If needed for the sake of giving a variety of nutrients, frozen organic fruits and vegetables (with nothing added) can be convenient and are a great way to have out-of-season foods all year.

 The best advice for new parents is to never stop feeding children the fruits and veggies they get as baby food. Don't stop when they start eating finger foods, or you'll never get them to eat broccoli when they're five.

Navigating the Toddler Years

My advice to any parent is to start their children on healthy, wholesome foods as young as possible. The younger they are, the more likely they are to know no different. However, if you wait until, say, preschool begins, you may find it challenging to introduce the plant-based foods you want your children to eat. The following sections outline some foods that you may not think to introduce. I also list some of the healthiest foods for toddlers and ideas about how to serve them.

Introducing a variety of foods

Toddlers (ages one to three) have gums that can "chew," and the enzyme production in their mouths has also become more active, so you can cut food into a size they can handle. Typically, a toddler requires approximately four to ten tablespoons a day of solid food, in addition to breast milk.

Here are some foods to introduce at this age:

- ✔ **Fruits (one to two servings per day):** Peaches, nectarines, melons, mangos, pineapples, plums, and papaya.

- ✔ **Veggies (one to two steamed servings per day):** Spinach, peppers, Swiss chard, turnips, onions, kale, asparagus, collards, eggplant, split peas, green peas, and lima beans.

- ✔ **Grains (six servings per day):** Quinoa, teff, rice, buckwheat, and millet. *Note:* You can try oats and barley after 15 months, and you can try wheat at 18 months, but watch for an allergy!

- ✔ **Legumes (¼ to ½ cup per day):** Kidney beans and chickpeas.

Gradually, you can add more foods, such as seeds (pumpkin and sunflower), amaranth, figs, raisins (soaked and pureed), lentils, beans, and tofu one to two times per week, and you can start introducing spices.

Choosing nutrient-dense foods

You can find so many wonderfully healthy options when it comes to feeding plant-based foods to your kid. You truly can't go wrong, but if you need a little help knowing where to start, here are some of the most nourishing plant-based foods for feeding your child in the early years.

- ✔ **Avocado:** Full of fiber, potassium, vitamin E, B vitamins, and folic acid, avocado is the ultimate nutrient-rich food. It's also sodium and cholesterol free. Per cup, avocado has 235 calories and 22 grams of fat — most of which is monounsaturated (the good kind).

  Avocado is super easy to serve. For infants, mash it up or scoop bites straight from the shell. For older children, make guacamole or drizzle slices with olive oil, balsamic vinegar, and a pinch of salt for a nutrient-rich salad.

- ✔ **Amaranth:** Most kids eat more than their fair share of white bread and pasta. If your child falls in the carb-loving camp, try serving him amaranth (a complex carbohydrate) instead. Compared to wheat, it has more calories, protein, and iron, and it has the most folic acid, calcium, and vitamin E of any grain.

  Amaranth seeds have a sweet, nutty flavor and can be popped like popcorn, added to soups or stews, and used to make hot cereal. It's also sold as flour and can be used to make healthy homemade bread.

- ✔ **Sweet potato:** Touted as one of the healthiest vegetables you can eat, sweet potatoes are complex carbohydrates that pack a nutritional punch. Rich in beta carotene, which the body converts to vitamin A, this root vegetable is easily digested and is a good source of vitamin C, potassium, and iron.

  Serve sweet potato puree (keep the skins on for additional nutrients), add cinnamon to spice it up, or mix with mashed bananas, pureed carrots, or applesauce. For children one year or older, roasted sweet potatoes make a great side dish, finger food, or on-the-go snack. Cut sweet potatoes into cubes and drizzle with olive oil, which adds healthy fats and calories, before roasting in a 350-degree oven for 45 minutes or until soft.

- ✔ **Blueberries:** Often referred to as a superfood, blueberries have more antioxidants — health-enhancing vitamins and enzymes — than any other fruit or vegetable. They're also high in fiber; just one cup delivers 14 percent of the daily recommended amount.

  Serve a bowl of blueberries as a snack; add them to muffins, pancakes, or fruit salads; or blend them with plain yogurt and ice for a nutrient-rich smoothie.

✔ **Lentils:** They may be small, but lentils pack a big nutritional punch. With 230 calories per cup, lentils have high levels of both soluble and insoluble fiber and are rich in iron and protein.

Mash up and blend lentils with pureed apples, sweet potatoes, or carrots.

✔ **Pumpkin seeds:** Compared to other seeds, the ones we dig out of our pumpkins each year — and often throw away — are among the most nutritious. A good source of magnesium (which strengthens nerves, muscles, and bones), pumpkin seeds contain immune-boosting zinc and a good amount of protein.

With 186 calories per ¼ cup, pumpkin seeds can add a sweet and nutty flavor to your child's favorite hot or cold cereal, yogurt, muffins, pancakes, or homemade granola. They're delicious on their own, too.

✔ **Nut butters:** Almonds are the healthiest nut of all. With 166 calories and 14 grams of fat in a one-ounce serving, almonds provide plenty of protein, fiber, calcium, zinc, iron, and vitamin E. However, if your child has a nut allergy, opt for sunflower-seed butter instead.

The best way to serve nut butters is on toast, on a sandwich, or as a dip for fruits and veggies.

Raising Healthy Kids and Teens

Kids and teens are potentially the most difficult age group to deal with when it comes to transitioning to healthier foods. That is, of course, if you didn't get them started young. Even if you did, you may find that with the influence of friends, school, and other groups they may join (such as sports or dance teams), they're exposed to all kinds of things you can't control.

The truth is, you don't have much control at this age (unless you want to be "that" parent). And if you do, your child may resist you, and you'll end up doing more damage than good. My suggestion is to just do your best to raise them on good principles and healthy eating and hope (with fingers crossed) that they make wise choices when it comes to food outside the home.

In the following sections, I offer some suggestions on how to help older kids give plant-based foods a chance. I also give you some ideas for guiding your kids through situations like eating lunch during the school day and attending birthday parties.

Overcoming resistance

There is no doubt that the more you push a lifestyle on your children, the more they may push back, and — at all costs — you want to avoid this resistance. You can take many approaches with your family to get everyone on board in a fun and innovative way that is "cool" enough for them to want to be part of it. Every family is unique, and there is no cookie-cutter approach to do this, so you may have to try a few different things to see what sticks.

Getting your kids involved

It's important that you get everyone involved in the process of preparing plant-based foods. Your kids are more likely to not only *try* new things but also be empowered or inspired to experiment and *create* their own recipes. Here are some suggestions for getting the whole family involved:

- ✔ Treat eating healthy as an exciting adventure. Make an experiment out of it and have your kids track the different tastes and preferences of everyone in the family.

- ✔ Have the kids help pick the recipes and get them involved with shopping and food prep. They're more likely to want to eat meals when they take part in or maybe even control the creation of them. You can even involve toddlers by offering them several healthy options and letting them select which foods they'd like to eat.

- ✔ Compromise with them — especially when they're younger than ten. Make up a chart of foods you know they like (for example, pizza and dessert). They can earn checks for trying new foods during the week, and when they've earned enough checks, you can make them a healthy version of their favorite food. This practice gets them to try things they wouldn't otherwise try and gives you peace of mind knowing they at least have some of the healthier food in their bellies.

- ✔ For older kids, show them the evidence about the benefits of eating a plant-based diet and let them make their own decisions. That way, you're not the enemy or unilaterally deciding for them.

- ✔ Encourage an interest in vegetables and fruits by growing a garden together and harvesting your own foods.

- ✔ Have a cooking challenge with the family (with judges!).

Compromising to make everyone happy

To make things work with your kids, you sometimes (read: often) have to compromise. For example, when you make a new recipe, always ask your kids to give it a fair chance with a positive attitude by trying at least one bite. If they don't care for it, let it be and don't force it on them. Of course, this approach can potentially create more resistance down the line when they figure out all they have to do is eat one bite and then get let off the hook. So instead of totally giving in, letting them have what they want, or making a whole other meal, make at least one thing at each meal that you know they do like, and let them have as much as they want. That way, everybody wins.

Another approach is to make the same recipe at least three or four times before you call it a wash. Sometimes the kids will come around, and sometimes they won't. Think of it this way: If you don't like to be asked to eat something you don't like, then don't do that to your kids.

If your child decides not to eat plant-based, don't freak out; just do your best to work with him. You may have to meet him halfway by letting him have his pick of some non-plant-based foods while still providing him with enough plant-based things that he'll eat. Remember, it doesn't have to be an all-or-nothing thing.

Speaking of that, why not let your kids have a "break" meal (or day)? In Chapter 5, I talk about different ways for adults to transition to a plant-based diet; you can adapt those same ideas to give your kids a break. Compromising is all about making sure everyone feels heard and "wins" a little something. You can find a happy medium!

Providing balanced meals and snacks

In our hectic lives, it can be difficult to always make and eat balanced meals and snacks. With school, extracurricular activities, and homework, your kids can easily miss out on proper nutrition. Here are some ideas to help you help your kids eat well:

- ✔ Whether you or your kids do it, pack lunches the day before. You already experience enough chaos in the morning, so pack the lunches the evening before.
- ✔ Also fill water bottles. Have them in the fridge, ready to tote.
- ✔ Cook things in batches that make good leftovers to take for lunch and heat up for future dinners.
- ✔ Pack plenty of fresh fruit in your kids' lunches, and make it *easy* for them to eat. Yes, it feels like a nuisance sometimes to peel those mandarins or cut oranges into bite-size pieces and pop them into a container. Why not just pack the whole fruit? Well, kids have very little time to eat in school, that's why. So, make it easy for them to eat that fruit. Peel and slice or cut into small pieces and pack in a container along with a fork. Kids are far more likely to eat it that way.

- Pack occasional treats — seaweed snacks, baked kale chips, and so on.

- Don't forget about weekends and after school! Have on hand plenty of healthy snacks that are ready to eat when hunger strikes.

- Keep sweet treats around, such as homemade muffins (see recipe in Chapter 10) or Apple Cinnamon Bites (see recipe in Chapter 14). They can be kept frozen and pulled out on demand for a delicious treat.

Handling occasions outside of your control

Although you get to be in control as a parent when kids are young, when your kids turn 12 or 13, look out! That's about the time when your children decide that *they* are in control. Add to that the situations they encounter outside of the house at school and with friends, and now you're even further removed. You have to find ways to work with these social situations that not only put you at ease but more importantly allow your children to make their own healthy decisions.

The school cafeteria and special events

Making a lunch for your child to take to school is the best way to avoid the cafeteria. If you make plentiful dinners at home, leftovers are the best bet. Other than that, you can create new lunches with your kids so they're excited about what they're taking and there are no surprises in their lunchboxes.

If your kids are on board with the plant-based lifestyle, then hopefully they won't let other kids or the food served at school influence them. This may be hard to believe, but I have many friends with kids who have proven this to be true. My advice is not to fall victim to what you think their influences are; don't serve them anything less than what you make at home.

If you're encountering some challenges or resistance from your child, be innovative with lunches so that your kid has something "cool" or comparable to what is served or what their friends may have.

Ultimately, you're trying to create healthy behaviors that will stay with your kids at any age. The goal is that they are satisfied with (and maybe even proud of) the food they eat so they don't feel deprived or embarrassed. If you're really lucky, they end up feeling like they have the best lunches ever!

Here are some healthy (and not embarrassing) foods you can try in your kids' lunches:

- A hearty sandwich
- Leftover pasta with tomato sauce
- Nori rolls (see recipe in Chapter 11)

✔ Baked yam fries and black-bean burger (see recipe in Chapter 12)

✔ Soba noodle salad (see recipe in Chapter 12)

Don't forget to add plant-based treats like cookies, muffins, and energy bites (see Chapter 13 for some great recipes).

If your kid eats school lunches and you're unhappy with what is being served, don't be afraid to address the school board. Maybe you even want to be part of the committee to help with advocating for healthier school lunches. Changes can be made to the system!

To preempt vending machine temptations, pack your kids a healthy plant-based chocolate bar or bag of chips once a week as a treat. First let them sample a few varieties at home to see what they like.

Birthday parties and sleepovers

Social situations call for a little bit of flexibility. Kids encounter many situations that challenge them (and you). Especially after you've spent years trying to mold their eating habits and palates, birthday parties, sleepovers, and other occasions present tempting treats. Your children may stick to their well-formed habits even when out, or (more likely) they'll have what their friends are having or what is being served. A lot of times, you have to just let these situations roll off your back and do the best you can, but here are some tips that can prevent some of this from happening:

✔ Try to make sure they eat something nourishing before going somewhere like a birthday party or sleepover.

✔ Encourage your children to participate in the *activities* at a party but not the food (especially if they're going on a full belly).

✔ Encourage them to select the plant-based options that are available (or, at the very least, the vegetarian options). If you're there with them, you can guide them.

✔ Send your children with their own food. Make sure to pick fun snacks that are similar to what is being offered so they don't feel left out. Maybe the other kids will even ask them what they're eating! However, first check with the party host to make sure none of the party guests is allergic to the food you're planning to send.

✔ Talk to the parents ahead of time to find out what they're serving or whether you can offer to make a few things for everyone to enjoy.

Once in a while, you may want to let your children eat what is offered — things like ice cream, cake, pizza, candy, fried chicken, and soda — so they can experience for themselves how they feel. They're more than likely to come home with a stomachache, which is their chance to see how their own choices impact them. It gives you a segue to talk about how unhealthy foods make you feel.

Hosting healthy Halloween celebrations

The best way to do Halloween is to do it in reverse! Instead of allowing your kids to go out and trick or treat on toxic (and most definitely *not* plant-based) candy, hand out healthier versions of snacks and treats at home while letting your kids make and eat healthy desserts like chocolate cake, cookies, and "ice cream" sundaes, all from natural, dairy-free sources. They can eat as much as they want, and you may notice that when you let them control with amounts, they actually stop sooner than you'd expect. Not to mention, that "healthy" dessert also has some nutrients (and not just empty calories).

Or, what about throwing a big plant-based Halloween party so your kids can invite friends over? It's a great way to help your kids not feel left out and introduce their friends to how "normal" this diet can be, *and* you know they're sticking to the menu!

Chapter 19

The Plant-Fueled Fitness Enthusiast

. . . .

In This Chapter

▶ Knowing which plants make the best fuel for an active body

▶ Understanding what to eat before, during, and after exercise

▶ Choosing the most natural supplements for fueling your body on the go

. . . .

*F*itness enthusiasts or just plain active individuals burn more energy than the average person, and if you're among them, you may be wondering whether you can stay properly fueled on plant-based foods alone. Don't fret, my athletic friend! It's possible to maintain proper fuel levels on plants alone. In fact, some of the world's most elite athletes swear by a plant-based diet.

Plants provide the necessary fuel for basic nutrition, and they can also be the source of the more-complex nutrition needed by individuals who take their physical activity to the next level. Fueling yourself on plant foods while engaging in athletic activity helps with performance, recovery, and much more.

In this chapter, I go through the ins and outs of eating properly while exercising, whether you're a fitness amateur or a serious athlete.

Boosting Macronutrients for the Active Person

The basic nutrients that we need to live healthfully are called macronutrients (see Chapter 3 for more info). Active people need exactly the same nutrients as average folks do, just usually in higher quantities, in certain ratios, and at certain times. An active person needs the perfect blend of all the major macros (proteins, carbs, and fats). Unfortunately, most of us are under the impression that active people need inordinate amounts of protein all the time, accompanied by pre-workout carb-loading. That's not really accurate, it turns out. Read on for more.

Plant-based protein for performance and recovery

Today's athletes (and the general population) have a misconception that we need to consume huge amounts of animal protein to gain muscle mass while losing fat. This isn't true. According to the World Health Organization, North Americans consume 100 to 200 grams of protein daily, which is enough for three to six people. The body can only absorb a certain amount of protein, and the rest is excreted as urine. So there's really no point in consuming more than your body can handle. Of course, those who are active may need somewhat higher amounts of protein, but eating a diet that is rich in plant protein can provide your body with more than enough.

Here are the top five plant proteins to eat if you're active:

- ✔ **Lentils:** For a plant-based fitness enthusiast, these are one of the best sources of protein, as they're rich in fiber and easy to digest. When cooked or sprouted, they're a rich source of protein (and even iron). They can be consumed in soup or stew, molded into a burger, or tossed into salads.

- ✔ **Spirulina:** Don't underestimate this blue-green algae, which comes from warm sources of fresh water. It's said to have more protein than red meat; it delivers 65 percent to 75 percent protein. It's also full of vital amino acids and minerals that are easily assimilated by the body. The best and easiest way for an active person to take spirulina is to add one teaspoon to one tablespoon (or three to five grams) to water, a smoothie, or juice.

- ✔ **Tempeh:** This happens to be one of my favorite sources of protein. Fermented, nutty, and full of texture, this plant protein is amazing for the athletic person and anyone plant-based because it's hearty and easy to digest. The best ways to enjoy tempeh are in a burger, in a stir-fry, or marinated and baked.

- ✔ **Quinoa:** This nutty seed is loaded with a full spectrum of amino acids and is brilliant for fitness gurus. It's the perfect post-workout recovery meal, as it's easy to digest and can be enjoyed for breakfast, lunch, or dinner.

- ✔ **Plant-based protein powder:** As long as it's a raw, sprouted plant protein, this definitely falls into the category of plant-powered proteins. It breaks down easily in liquids and makes amazing smoothies. Be sure to select a powder that's sourced from rice, hemp, or pea.

For more sources of protein, see Chapter 3.

Protein *builds* muscle; it doesn't *fuel* muscle. So protein is better eaten post-workout. Eating too much protein before intense exercise can result in muscle cramping. This is because protein requires more fluid in order to be metabolized than do carbohydrates or fat, and cramping occurs when the body isn't properly hydrated. Protein also creates toxins when it's burned, which puts unwanted stress on the body during exercise, leading to a decline in endurance.

Functional fats

The body needs fats for every function. If our cells aren't thriving and functioning optimally, then our bodies won't either, and that spells disaster, especially if you're active. The energy that one gram of fat provides can be profound in terms of performance. As I detail in Chapter 3, there are *essential fats* and *non-essential fats*. The ones our body can't produce on its own (essential fats) need to be derived from our diet.

The top five plant-based foods that provide essential fats are:

- ✔ **Avocado:** Containing a wide array of nutrients, including omega 3s, protein, and vitamin E, this perfect food provides the necessary sustenance for an active person who is burning a lot of energy. It can be spread on toast for a nourishing, quick, and easy-to-eat snack on the go.

- ✔ **Coconut oil:** Coconut oil is one of the best oils for athletes and for weight loss. The medium-chain fats in coconut oil provide long and sustained energy before a workout and also help with inflammation and recovery after a workout. The body can break it down and assimilate it quite rapidly. It provides the body with efficient energy, which means it's burned as energy more quickly than it gets stored as fat. It can be scooped into a smoothie, spread on toast, or eaten by the spoonful for a burst of energy or to help with recovery after a workout.

- ✔ **Chia seeds:** These teeny seeds pack an incredible punch and provide the body with so much energy that you wonder why more people don't eat them more often. They're loaded with higher levels of omega-3 fatty acids than any other plant source. They're great for endurance and recovery. They also have antioxidants and potassium. They can be soaked to make a breakfast cereal or added to smoothies, salads, soups, and energy cookies.

- ✔ **Almonds:** These classic nuts offer the most protein, fiber, and vitamin E of all the nuts. They contain monounsaturated fats, which are good for reducing inflammation after a hard training session. Almonds can be added to trail mix, smoothies, or cereal or snacked on alone. Organic almond butter is also a tasty option once in a while to spread on toast or stir into chia pudding or oatmeal.

✔ **Hempseeds:** These little seeds act as both fat and protein, making hempseeds one of the best sources of plant protein and fat. They contain protein, fiber, B vitamins, vitamin E, and the highest level of essential fats of all seeds. They also make an excellent milk or salad topper and are delicious in smoothies and cereals. Your body has to do very little work to break them down, and they're good for muscle building and recovery.

Carbs for the mind and body

Carbohydrates, which fuel the body, are essential for optimal performance. But don't be too hasty; although your muscles need those carbs to burn, it's all about eating the *right kind* of carbs — that is, complex carbs (for more on carbs, see Chapter 3).

Your body naturally craves complex carbs for sustained energy. Don't ignore these cravings! Complex carbs are our bodies' preferred source of energy (over simple carbs, protein, or fat). To make sure you're getting enough energy for your activity level, eat a variety of fruits, whole-grain pastas and breads, and vegetables, and eat these complex carbs in small doses throughout the day to ensure optimum glycogen storage.

Here are the top five plant-based complex carbs for athletes:

✔ **Sweet potatoes:** The slow-burning source of energy that sweet potatoes provide is amazing for athletes. The sugars in sweet potatoes are low on the glycemic index and full of vitamin A and antioxidants. They soothe sore muscles and maintain fluids in the body. They can be baked into french fries; shredded into burgers; and chopped into soups, stews, and stir-fries.

✔ **Wild rice:** This grass is more diverse and nutritious than brown rice because it contains both protein and fiber. It's also gluten free, high in fiber, and easy to break down. It's a great source of vitamins A, C, and E, along with zinc and potassium. This makes it a nutritional powerhouse for a moving body and a great post-workout meal. Wild rice can be eaten in salad and tastes amazing in soups.

✔ **Oats:** They're the perfect heart-healthy breakfast grain — high in fiber and low in saturated fat. They contain magnesium, which helps maintain nerve and muscle function and metabolic reactions in the body. Have some for breakfast or load it into a power bar or muffin.

✔ **Bananas:** Bananas contain not only potassium that helps restore nerve and muscle function (which is what they're known for in the athletic world) but also vitamin C. They help support the immune system and contain prebiotics that help maintain healthy bacteria in your gut. They provide a quick natural source of energy and sugar and make the perfect snack for a busy body (not to be confused with a busybody). Smoothies, cereals, cookies, and desserts are a few great places for bananas.

✔ **Chickpeas:** Chickpeas provide a good amount of complex carbohydrates per cup, as well as protein and fiber. The slow, steady release of carbs helps to balance blood-sugar levels over long periods of high activity. They're great for dips, in salads and soups, or even just to snack on.

For the most part, avoid foods with a high glycemic index, such as corn, white potatoes, instant cereals, white rice, white breads, and other refined foods. They raise your blood sugar and insulin levels rapidly.

Eating Before and After Workouts

Eating the right foods before and after workouts is essential to performance and recovery. Often, people neglect this important aspect of nutrition. Plant-based food sources are diverse enough that many can be eaten either before or after workouts. Here's a closer look at some specific foods for pre- and post-workout dining.

Eating before your workout

The most important thing to consider for a pre-workout snack is its digestibility: You want to eat simple foods that require little energy to break down. Less blood going to digestion means more blood for your muscles. This reduces your chances of getting a cramp in your diaphragm because of undigested food. Making sure you're adequately hydrated pre-workout is also key. This decreases the amount of stress on the body and allows it to work harder and perform better, resulting in less recovery time.

Your first choice for fuel before intense exercise should be complex carbohydrates. They provide sustained, long-lasting energy release. Choose sources that your body can digest easily and efficiently. This way, your energy is primarily directed to your workout. Choose from sources such as dried fruit, fresh fruit, sprouted whole-grain bread, whole-grain pasta, and oatmeal.

Your pre-workout meal should also be determined by the length of your workout and the level of intensity.

✔ **High-intensity short workouts** (less than an hour of short, intense work, such as sprints, interval training, jumping rope, and cross fit) require food that goes straight to the liver for immediate energy because there's no time for conversion or digestion. Examples include dates, figs, fruit, and coconut oil. Consume food 30 to 60 minutes before activity.

✔ **Medium-intensity workouts** (one to two hours), such as 10-kilometer runs, half marathons, endurance swimming, step classes, power hiking, power yoga, and long-distance cycling, should be fueled by small amounts of alkaline protein, such as raw hemp, and essential fatty acids, such as ground flaxseeds or chia seeds, for prolonged energy and improved endurance. Consume food one to two hours before activity.

✔ **Low-intensity workouts** (one to two hours), such as long hikes, light jogging, Pilates, recreational swimming, and basketball, should be fueled by pre-workout snacks that have three times more carbohydrates than fat and protein. During this type of exercise, the body primarily burns fat, but your body burns muscle if not enough amino acids are present even for a short time in the fat-burning zone. Hence the need to consume a small amount of protein before a long exercise period. It also slows the release of carbohydrates, leading to improved endurance, preventing muscle loss, and keeping body fat to a minimum. Consume food one to two hours before activity.

✔ **Strenuous, long-duration workouts,** such as triathlons and marathons (and any endurance activities lasting longer than two to three hours), should be fueled by a combination of complex carbohydrates, fat, and protein to prolong endurance and slow the release of energy from the liver. Check out my recipe for Apple Cinnamon Energy Bites in Chapter 14. Consume food one and a half to three hours before activity.

Now that you know *what* to eat, knowing *when* to eat these foods is just as important. Depending on the length of your workout, you want to fuel yourself accordingly; here's a sample timeline and menu for your pre-workout food regimen:

1. **One hour or more before a workout:** Eat one to two slices of sprouted or whole-grain bread with almond butter, one cup of soaked oats, or Super Chia Banana Porridge (see recipe in Chapter 10).

2. **Thirty minutes to one hour before a workout:** Try a piece of fruit, a few dates, a handful of trail mix, or a small piece of a homemade energy bar (see recipe for Brown-Rice Krispy Bars in Chapter 14).

3. **Thirty minutes or fewer before a short workout:** Have coconut water with green powder, a tablespoon of coconut oil, or half an apple.

Eating during your workout

It's critically important to replenish your body during long, intense, or sustained workouts. Activities such as running, cycling, and triathlons require you to continually take in quick, easy energy so the body can stay fueled and perform effectively.

Because the body is working hard while exercising and focusing on delivering nutrients to working muscles, it can only handle so much. Choosing foods that are easy to both eat and digest is extremely important. And remember, they also have to travel well.

Think of marathoners and long-distance cyclists. Heavy foods take up too much space in their packs and require too much energy to digest, so these athletes need on-the-go fuel that is easily accessible. If you're an endurance athlete, choose things like dried fruits (dates, figs, and apricots are great choices), energy bars, nuts, or even homemade energy gel (see sidebar).

For longer activities (two or more hours) that aren't as intense as cycling or running — something like hiking, swimming, or team sports like tennis, hockey, or baseball — lean lightly on the quick energy and more heavily on more-complex snacks. An energy bar, trail mix with nuts and seeds, whole-grain muffin, or smoothie can be consumed midway for the nutrition the body needs to carry on performing.

Refueling post-workout

The 45-minute period immediately following a workout is referred to as the *fuel window*. Within that window, muscles are better able to absorb the carbohydrates in food and convert them into fuel, which speeds up recovery time. You should aim to have a post-workout snack that contains carbs, fats, and proteins. Yes, it should even contain some simple sugars (such as honey, maple syrup, or fruit), because you need the quick energy to get nutrients into your muscles. The protein component helps rebuild and repair your muscles, and the fat helps reduce inflammation and speed up recovery.

Homemade energy gel

Whip up a batch of this energy gel when you want some nutritious, easily portable fuel for long or intense workouts.

2 dates

1 tablespoon honey or coconut nectar

2 tablespoons ground or whole chia seeds

1 tablespoon cacao powder

1 tablespoon coconut oil

Blend together into a gel consistency. Place in a small bag or container that can be accessed easily during a workout.

If you have a regular workout schedule but aren't training hard, eating fresh fruit after exercise is a good way to balance your blood-sugar levels. If the workout is notably draining, such as a spin class or other high-intensity work, your best option is a liquid meal, such as a smoothie. Eating a full meal after a workout requires a large amount of blood to travel to the stomach to aid in digestion. This takes away from its delivery of nutrients to the extremities of the body, and recovery can dramatically decrease.

About an hour after your post-workout snack, consume a complete nutrient-rich meal that includes high-quality and easily digestible protein, omega-3 fats, vitamins, and minerals from plant-based sources. Post-workout meals should include protein to help build and repair muscle. But don't make your meal just protein — although it prevents muscle loss, too much protein after a workout can slow down recovery. In addition to protein, your body needs a small amount of carbs for support after working out. Carbs help support recovery and growth without shutting off the fat-burning process.

Checking out the chocolate-milk craze

Chocolate dairy milk is being marketed as the perfect post-workout food. For recovery and replenishment, it shows up in gyms and health magazines, and more people are buying into it. Unfortunately, this drink, which is loaded with sugar and fake chocolate, isn't the perfect post-workout food. Sure, it provides the body with the calories and carbohydrates required after a heavy workout, but not the right kind.

Chocolate dairy milk obviously doesn't fit into a plant-based diet, and it's also extremely hard on the body. Dairy requires a lot of energy to digest, and after a workout your body may not have that much energy available. Also, dairy milk is acidic; because the body is already in an acidic state after a workout, dairy milk can actually slow recovery. And dairy milk can stimulate an increase in mucus, which can hinder breathing all day but especially during exercise.

Instead, I suggest a delicious whole-food alternative that meets the same criteria for calories and carbohydrates. I call it Marni's Perfect Chocolate Recovery Shake.

2 cups non-dairy milk (rice, almond, or coconut)

1 scoop plant-based protein powder (hemp or brown-rice based)

1 to 2 tablespoons pure cacao powder

Mix the ingredients together in a glass jar, shaker cup, or water bottle.

When you drink this, you won't notice a huge difference in taste from chocolate dairy milk (other than that it tastes more pure), but the effect on your body and how it recovers is extremely different. Whichever non-dairy milk you choose, you get a boost of carbohydrates, protein, and fat — easy-to-digest protein from the powder and magnesium and antioxidants from the pure cacao — all of which nourish your cells post workout.

For an amazing post-workout meal, try a protein-rich Happy Hemp Loaf or a Chocolate Banana Super Smoothie (see recipes in Chapter 14).

 Don't skip your post-workout meal! Skipping food after a long workout leads to shakiness for the rest of the day and lethargy during your next workout. It may cause you to miss workouts, and it may cause your body to raise cortisol levels, retain body fat, and cannibalize muscle tissue.

Sorting Out Supplements: Sports Drinks, Energy Bars, and Protein Powders

Sports supplements are a key addition to any active person's diet. They provide a convenient way to get more protein, minerals, and other nutrients into your meals. However, it's crucial that the ingredients are clean, natural, and as simple as possible. Let's sort out the good from the gross.

Sports drinks

One of the most popular drinks in North America, sports drinks make electrolytes readily available. The nutrients they provide are important to avoid cramping, *hyponatremia* (an electrolyte imbalance that occurs when a person drinks too much water), muscle twitches, heart palpitations, and loss of consciousness. Dehydration can disturb the delicate electrolyte balance that is essential for all bodily functions, and sports drinks help maintain this balance.

However, the ones typically available in stores contain artificial colors and flavors and are loaded with refined sugar, none of which have a place in proper hydration. Many sports drinks on the market are simply flavored sugar water marketed with a sporty image. You don't need vitamins or carbonation in a sports drink. Also, be sure to avoid preservatives!

So what are your options? Well, my preferred option is coconut water, which has been used by the professional Brazilian soccer team for several decades. It's rich in electrolytes and can help maintain smooth muscle contractions and energy levels.

 Drink coconut water slightly chilled, as this allows for better absorption (and tastes better). Don't forget to drink beyond your thirst to rehydrate!

Seaweeds (dulse in particular) also have a nicely balanced electrolyte profile that you can include in your water to make your own sports drinks and energy bars.

What you need are the two main electrolytes: sodium and potassium. Having both sodium (the major electrolyte you lose when you sweat) and potassium is important because both nutrients help with fluid absorption and retention, as well as promoting proper nerve conduction for the optimal firing of your muscles when exercising.

Energy bars

Energy bars are a great way to get a properly balanced serving of all the right nutritional elements you need for an effective and safe workout. But just like anything, some options are better than others. Here are five things to look for when shopping for energy bars:

- ✔ A natural protein source, such as nuts, seeds, quinoa, brown-rice protein, or hemp protein
- ✔ Natural sweeteners, such as brown-rice syrup, honey, maple syrup, or coconut nectar
- ✔ A short ingredient list with ingredients you recognize
- ✔ Less sugar than a typical candy bar (24 grams of sugar)
- ✔ As few processed ingredients as possible

When in doubt, go for the bars that are composed of nuts and seeds, but remember to check the sweetener.

Protein powders

Protein powder is great, not only to ensure that your muscles are repaired but also to meet your daily protein needs if you live a busy, on-the-go lifestyle as a plant-based eater. Unfortunately, many popular protein powders include cheap fillers, artificial colors, and artificial sweeteners that are simply unnecessary. Cheap protein powders can actually harm your recovery by causing your body to become acidic. Instead, use plant-based protein to bring your body back into an alkalized state and repair your muscles after a workout.

Brown-rice protein and hemp protein are your best bets. Skip soy protein, which is often of poor quality and made with genetically modified ingredients. The isolated form of soy protein is difficult to digest and is extremely processed, whereas hemp and brown-rice proteins are typically used in their raw form — sprouted, germinated, and milled to extract the protein without heat. (This keeps the proteins intact.)

Aside from after workouts, protein powder makes a great afternoon snack to curb cravings and balance blood-sugar levels. Shake it up with a cup of rice or almond milk.

Ingredients to avoid

Now that you know the good ingredients to look for in packaged supplements, it's time to expose the gross ingredients that are lurking in many packaged supplements that you want to avoid putting in your body:

- ✔ **High-fructose corn syrup:** This inexpensive sweetener is worse than regular white sugar. It's the most processed form of sugar, is genetically modified, and may cause insulin resistance and a slew of other health problems.

- ✔ **Soy protein isolate:** It may sound natural and healthy, being a soy product and all, but it's not something you can make yourself, which is the first red flag. It's put through several acidic and alkalizing baths to remove fiber and separate and neutralize it. It's also processed at high temperatures that can change the structure of some of the proteins.

- ✔ **Whey protein:** The most popular protein out there isn't as great as many people assume. Although it does have a high absorption rate in the body, it's also extremely allergenic. It doesn't contain lactose, but because it's still a dairy product it can cause mild allergic reactions, such as inflammation and bloating.

- ✔ **Natural flavors:** You may think that "natural flavors" equals healthy, but this ingredient is usually MSG. Commonly found in takeout meals, MSG is a flavor enhancer that can cause side effects like facial pressure, headaches, nausea, and chest pains. If you see "natural flavors" on a package, contact the company and ask it to identify its sources of these flavors.

- ✔ **Fractioned palm oil:** This cheap oil is used for its high heat stability. It's bleached, filtered, melted, degummed, and refined before it's ever added to a food product. Look out for palm-kernel oil, as well, as it can't be obtained naturally; it has to be extracted from the pit with gasoline-like solvent.

- ✔ **Maltodextrin:** Another corn product finds its way into our food with this cheap, easily digestible sweetener. It is low-calorie and absorbed as quickly as regular glucose. It is nowhere near a natural product, and it's genetically modified.

✓ **Artificial sweeteners:** Common sweeteners found in "health-food" products are maltitol and sucralose. Maltitol is a low-calorie hydrogenated maltose made from genetically modified cornstarch. Sucralose is calorie-free chlorinated sugar. The problem with these low- or zero-calorie products is that their sweetness tricks the body into thinking it's receiving some form of energy (sugar). When the body only receives a chemical sweetener, its craving for energy isn't satisfied, and you end up craving more sugar.

Following the Vitamin and Mineral Code

Specific micronutrients, such as calcium, iron, vitamin B12, vitamin C, vitamin D, and zinc, are required when you're active and on a plant-based diet (head to Chapter 3 for more on micronutrients). These vitamins and minerals are essential components of a vegetarian or vegan diet, so it's important to get them through a variety of sources. Luckily, the plant-based world offers lots of vitamin- and mineral-rich foods; however, some essential vitamins may require minimal supplementation.

Exercising is all about breaking your system down and building it back up, so it's vital that you get enough of these:

✓ **Calcium:** Bone health is key to overall health and fitness. If your bones aren't strong enough, they can't support your daily activities. As you know, you can build strong bones with calcium-rich foods, such as leafy greens, root veggies, almonds, sesame seeds, legumes, and fermented soy. And avoiding animal products altogether can help your body hold on to the circulating calcium it already has.

✓ **Iron:** Yes, you can get iron from plants! Iron is essential for the blood, circulation, liver function, immunity, and maintaining protein and enzymes in the body. Iron in plant-based foods is actually better on a per-calorie basis than meat. Iron absorption is increased especially when eating foods containing vitamin C. Iron can be found in dark leafy greens, blackstrap molasses, kidney beans, chickpeas, tempeh, beet greens, tahini, peas, raisins, millet, and kale.

✓ **Zinc:** Zinc is a mineral that helps in the healing of wounds and is an antioxidant. It also stabilizes membranes, synthesizes collagen, and reduces inflammation. It's readily available in many plant foods, such as whole grains (bread, pasta, and rice), wheat germ, tofu, tempeh, millet, quinoa, miso, legumes, sprouts, nuts, and seeds.

✔ **Vitamin C:** Most fruits and vegetables are bursting with this super antioxidant vitamin. Vitamin C is essential for tissue growth and repair, immunity, energy, and cell regeneration, and it helps the body ward off oxidative stress. Taking vitamin C after working out can be helpful for proper recovery. Essential sources of vitamin C are oranges, grapefruit, lemons, strawberries, broccoli, kiwi, peppers, and Brussels sprouts.

✔ **Vitamin B12:** Although the requirement for B12 is very low, it can be difficult to get from a plant-based diet. B12 is essential for the blood and nervous system. Because of its role in blood-cell production, B12 is crucial for plant-based athletes, as it helps get oxygen into your tissues. Luckily, you can try various plant-based sources, such as nutritional yeast, tempeh, miso, and seaweed. You may also need to take a B12 supplement, preferably in methylcobalamin form.

✔ **Vitamin D:** Athletes and active individuals require adequate vitamin D to maintain bone health, improve immunity, and boost overall physical performance. Vitamin D is one of the only vitamins that can't be obtained from a plant-based diet. But the good news is that as long as you get some sunlight every day, you can more than replenish your vitamin D stores. If you live in a climate with little sunshine, you may want to consider plant-based supplementation.

✔ **Omega-3 fatty acids:** Omega-3 fats are essential for energy production and brain function, as well as tissue repair and regeneration and blood circulation. Some plant-based sources include flaxseeds, flaxseed oil, chia seeds, chia oil, hempseeds, avocados, walnuts, and sprouted tofu. It's important to note, however, that oils like flaxseed oil and chia oil aren't as wholesome as the seeds themselves. It's okay to use them on occasion, but be sure to buy organic varieties packaged in dark bottles. And buy small quantities, because these oils don't last very long after they're opened.

Chapter 20

Getting Older, Getting Wiser about Your Plant-Based Diet

*G*rowing older can be fraught with unwelcome changes: Your body isn't as strong as it once was, you may develop a lifelong or life-altering condition or disease, or you may not have as much energy as you once did. For those reasons, you want to make sure that everything you consume is good for you; there's no room for error at this stage. As you age, your body doesn't handle junk food or heavy foods the same way it did when you were younger, so it's critical to know the nutrients you need and to avoid foods that don't contribute to your well-being.

The physiological changes that occur with aging alter nutrient needs. As a result, packing more nutrition into fewer calories becomes a challenge for older adults, which means you must focus on quality food choices. The senior population can really benefit from a plant-based diet. This chapter outlines the positive effects a plant-based diet can have on older folks.

Knowing How Plants Contribute to a Longer Life

Eating more plants can lead to a longer life. The power they have to prevent disease and boost immunity and overall health is just amazing. In the following sections, I provide you with some of the research that proves the remarkable benefits of following a plant-based diet as you age.

Pondering how plants protect your cells

Sometimes a little hard research is all it takes to prove (or at least highlight) a point. People who follow a plant-based diet are generally less prone to obesity and disease. A small pilot study concluded in 2013 found that switching to a health-conscious diet and lifestyle can actually reverse cell aging.

The Preventive Medicine Research Institute and the University of California, San Francisco, conducted a study of 35 men in their 50s and 60s. Ten of the men switched for five years to a mostly vegan diet rich in plant-based protein, fruits, vegetables, unrefined grains, and legumes. They also exercised for a minimum of 30 minutes a day, six days a week, and did some type of stress management (such as meditation, yoga, or stretching) for an hour every day.

At the end of the five-year study, the 10 men who made healthy lifestyle changes showed a 10 percent lengthening of their cells' telomeres, implying that the cells would have a longer life span. The 25 men who hadn't made any lifestyle changes showed a 3 percent shortening in cell telomeres. The study indicates that by making lifestyle changes such as exercising, shifting to a plant-based diet, and reducing stress, you can increase the relative length of telomeres, which are the parts of chromosomes that impact cell aging.

Eating a plant-based diet lowers your risk for some chronic diseases and health conditions, including heart disease, diabetes, and some forms of cancer, according to the Boston University School of Public Health. People who eat a plant-based diet also tend to exercise more and smoke less than omnivores (people who include animal-based products in their diet).

Understanding telomeres

Telomeres are the sequences at the end of a chromosome that protect that chromosome from deterioration. During chromosome replication, the enzymes that duplicate DNA can't continue the duplication all the way to the end of the chromosome, so in each duplication the end of the chromosome is shortened. The telomeres are disposable buffers that protect the genes on the chromosome from being cut off. With each cell division, the telomere ends become shorter. The small study I mention in this chapter, conducted by the Preventive Medicine Research Institute and the University of California, San Francisco, shows that a plant-based diet can help lengthen telomeres, giving cells a longer life span, although larger studies are needed to confirm this finding.

Slowing down diseases

These days, it sometimes seems like a given that we're all going to contract some major disease or health condition. Many seniors suffer from myriad health problems, but if you're a plant-based eater, you may be able to avoid or reverse some of the conditions of aging.

Convincing evidence shows that plant-based diets can slow, prevent, and treat numerous chronic diseases, including heart disease, hypertension, stroke, cancer, obesity, diabetes, gallbladder disease, arthritis, kidney disease, gastro-intestinal disorders, and asthma.

There are several reasons for this. Plant-based eaters:

- ✓ Tend not to be overweight compared to non-plant-based eaters.

- ✓ Consume less saturated fat. (Saturated fat may increase insulin secretion, potentially leading to insulin insensitivity, a cause of diabetes.)

- ✓ Consume much higher amounts of fiber (especially soluble fiber), which improves blood-glucose response in the blood, which is linked to diabetes and obesity.

- ✓ Consume more magnesium. (Insufficient magnesium may lead to insulin resistance, which can lead to diabetes.)

- ✓ Consume more unrefined foods, such as whole grains, legumes, vegetables, nuts, and seeds. (These foods help improve digestion and gut health because of their fiber and help keep our cells strong and healthy.)

- ✓ Consume a lot of foods that are rich in antioxidants, which are powerful protectors against free-radical damage and are linked to a reduced risk of cataracts, macular degeneration, heart disease, various forms of cancer, and even wrinkles.

If you want specifics, here are some common health conditions that many individuals, including seniors, face and details about how a plant-based diet can slow or reverse them:

- ✓ **Heart disease and high cholesterol:** In North America, heart disease accounts for about 40 percent of all deaths. Of all dietary groups, plant-based eaters have the lowest intakes of saturated fat, trans fatty acids, and cholesterol, all of which are bad for your heart. The most powerful cholesterol-lowering agents are soluble fiber, plant protein, polyunsaturated fats, and phytochemicals, all of which are found exclusively or primarily in plant foods. It comes as no surprise that plant-based eaters have the lowest total and LDL cholesterol levels of all dietary groups.

- ✔ **Cancer:** Experts estimate that improving diet and exercise alone could prevent 30 percent to 40 percent of all cancers. Vegetable and fruit consumption, in addition to the elimination of animal products, is associated with a lower risk of almost all types of cancer.

- ✔ **Obesity:** Heart disease and hypertension are both associated with excessive body weight. A plant-based diet can keep weight in check because of its high fiber content (which improves satiety), lower fat content (which reduces caloric density), and higher glucagon secretion (glucagon increases blood-glucose concentration, promotes appetite control, and increases fat oxidation).

- ✔ **Diabetes:** Diabetes is the seventh-leading cause of death in the United States. Approximately 80 percent of those suffering from type 2 diabetes are overweight. Excess body weight is the single most important risk factor for type 2 diabetes. Worldwide, the lowest frequency of type 2 diabetes is found among populations eating plant-based diets.

- ✔ **Strokes:** Plant-based eaters have a reduced risk for stroke because of their high-fiber, low-saturated-fat, cholesterol-free, phytochemical-rich diets.

- ✔ **High blood pressure:** The risk of both coronary artery disease and stroke is increased by high blood pressure. Although plant-based populations have slightly lower blood pressures than non-vegetarians, rates of hypertension are even lower because of a diet higher in fiber, potassium, magnesium, and phytochemicals; lower in total and saturated fat consumption; and possibly lower in sodium intake.

Ensuring You're Getting the Right Nutrients

As you age, it becomes even more important to make sure you're getting the most nutritional mileage out of every bite and sip. And that starts with making sure you're eating the right foods and avoiding ones that lack nutrients and contain empty calories.

Getting enough of special nutrients

As we age, we need to pay greater attention to and make a bigger effort to get enough of certain nutrients. Of course, which vitamins and minerals are critical depends on the health status of each individual, but some of the most important are:

✔ **Calcium:** As we age, our bodies don't absorb calcium as easily as they once did. Increased calcium excretion accompanies decreased absorption. Age-associated loss of bone density increases the risk for fractures and osteoporosis. The loss of skeletal calcium in postmenopausal women can reach more than 40 percent. Because bone fractures are a significant contributor to morbidity and mortality in older people, achieving daily calcium needs is critical, yet only 5 percent of older women and 10 percent of older men consume the daily recommended amount (1,200 micrograms per day). Make sure you get yours!

✔ **Vitamin D:** Evidence suggests that vitamin D, best known for its role in bone health, may have a function in preventing a number of diseases. According to dietary guidelines, the need for the "sunshine vitamin" increases from 15 micrograms to 20 micrograms per day after age 70 as blood levels of vitamin D decline. For the elderly, higher amounts (20 micrograms per day) from both fortified foods and supplements are recommended.

✔ **Vitamin B12 and folate:** Most individuals over age 50 have a reduced ability to absorb naturally occurring B12 and must therefore consume it in its crystalline form (through fortified foods or supplements). Vitamin B12 deficiency can cause cognitive dysfunction and neurological problems in older people.

✔ **Sodium:** Because many people develop hypertension at some point during their lifetime — typically, the higher their salt intake, the higher their blood pressure — older adults should aim to consume no more than 1,500 milligrams of sodium per day (about ¾ teaspoon of sea salt). As a group, older adults tend to be more salt sensitive than others.

✔ **Fiber:** Because constipation may affect up to 20 percent of people over age 65, foods rich in dietary fiber become increasingly important for older adults. Additional causes of constipation among this age group may include side effects of medications and lack of appropriate hydration. Low fiber intake may also contribute to other gastrointestinal diseases common among older adults, including diverticulosis.

✔ **Adequate fluid intake:** Drinking enough fluids not only eases constipation; it also helps avert dehydration, a serious threat to the elderly. Causes of impaired fluid and electrolyte balance include physiological impairments in renal function and thirst perception, reduced body fluid, and blunted medication effects. Severe dehydration in the elderly can lead to cognitive impairment and functional decline.

✔ **Other nutrients:** The role of antioxidants in the aging process is worth mentioning. Zinc, along with vitamins C and E and the phytochemicals lutein, zeaxanthin, and beta carotene from food sources, may help prevent or slow the onset of age-related macular degeneration, the leading cause of blindness in people over age 55.

Figuring out nutrition shakes

Nutrition drinks (sold under names like Ensure and Boost) have become the go-to "healthy" drink for the elderly population (and even for younger people who are in a compromised state of digestion or who aren't getting a full spectrum of nutrients). However, I must caution that these well-marketed milkshakes contain low-quality ingredients, including milk powder, sugar, and preservatives.

The marketers of these nutritional drinks claim that these products meet all of your nutrition requirements in one beverage, but this is far from the truth. With ingredients like corn, maltodextrin, milk protein, and canola oil, these products aren't even plant-based! They can actually be harmful to your health, causing gas, bloating, constipation, and — in some cases — rashes and other discomforts.

The good news is that there's an easy solution. You can make your own well-rounded beverages from protein powders based on brown rice or hemp. These are easy to digest and absorb and can be blended with non-dairy milks for an easy drink to sip. Check out Chapters 10 and 14 for some healthy smoothie ideas.

Training caregivers on the plant-based approach

If you have limited mobility, you may rely on someone else to do your grocery shopping or deliver or prepare your meals. Maybe a relative or a caregiver helps with your meals. Yet you still want to stick to your plant-based diet. So how do you make sure you get the foods you want? Here are some tips for making sure other folks understand the importance of buying and preparing plant-based foods for you:

- ✔ If needed, conduct thorough interviews so you can select a trained caretaker or live-in aide who can shop for, prepare, and cook plant-based healthy meals that are wholesome. Don't settle for someone who doesn't support or understand this diet.

- ✔ Research different food-delivery services that can customize or provide healthy meals or fresh groceries to your door. Many seniors use Meals on Wheels, but if you've got some extra funds, you can find many fresh, box-based food-delivery services. Make sure to inquire about their plant-based menus before committing to a service. Don't be afraid to stand up for yourself (or get a loved one to make the call for you).

✔ Keep your eyes and ears open for other plant-based seniors who are in a similar situation and find out what they do, or maybe team up with them for group meals or recipe exchanges.

✔ If someone else does your shopping, give him or her a crash course on how to navigate nutrition labels (see Chapter 8 for a refresher).

Preparing plant-based foods for easier consumption

Traditional chewing may become more difficult over the years. Mouths, teeth, and metabolism all change. Often, the way we crunched or munched on a salad or sandwich in the past may no longer be appealing or physiologically possible. Dental decay, swollen gums, improperly fitted dentures, reduced salivation, impaired oral control resulting from stroke and dementia, and loss of appetite can plague the elderly population, but we can always take a softer approach.

The preparation of textured, modified foods by way of mincing and pureeing may minimize the amount of chewing necessary while allowing you to maintain adequate nutrient intake.

It's entirely possible to get excellent nutrition on a soft-food or "cut up" diet. If eating crunchy fruits and vegetables is difficult, try softer options. Use ripe fruits, such as papaya, peaches, nectarines, mangos, pears, bananas, melons, kiwi, and berries. You may also find cooked or steamed vegetables easier to eat, so try soft-cooked squash, yams, sweet potatoes, zucchini, eggplant, potatoes, and other veggies, and don't forget about a nicely marinated or seasoned serving of tofu. Here's a quick list of plant-based soft foods:

✔ Steamed or cooked vegetables

✔ Soft, ripe fruits

✔ Fruit purees

✔ Fruit or green smoothies

✔ Homemade vegetable juices

✔ Applesauce

✔ Soft grains, such as porridge (see the recipe in Chapter 10)

✔ Soft proteins, such as tofu or pureed or blended beans

✔ Vegetable soup purees

Invest in a good juicer, blender and/or food processor so you can easily make nutritious juice blends and pureed foods at home.

Working with Prescriptions and Diet

Your diet accounts for most of the health benefits you reap from a healthy lifestyle, so staying on (or even starting) a plant-based diet throughout your senior years can make a huge positive impact — naturally.

Members of the aging population are often on at least one prescription drug. Doctors prescribe medications for seniors at an alarmingly high rate. And although *some* of these medications are no doubt warranted, many are not. Unfortunately, this over-reliance on medication has taken a toll on seniors' health. Consider how many times a prescribed pill causes another ailment or condition as a side effect, prompting the doctor to prescribe another pill, and it turns into a vicious cycle.

Over the years, this perpetual medicating can drastically age someone and cause more harm than good. Although I'm in no position to tell anyone to stop taking her medications, I do suggest that the more you work with your diet to increase the nutrients you get from whole foods, the more likely it is that you'll boost your health naturally. The good news is that, in time, you and your doctor may find that you can gradually wean off of the pills you thought you would have to take for the rest of your life.

Taking fewer pills, getting more health

If you want to live a long and healthy life, avoiding drugs as much as possible — even those that are prescribed to you — is a good idea. Of course, you need to consult with your health-care provider if you choose to go this route.

You don't typically expect your medications to harm you, as they're usually prescribed for a reason. However, be mindful that taking drugs, especially painkillers or multiple drugs, can pose greater risks to your health than sitting behind the wheel of a car.

Now, I'm not telling you to throw all your pills out the window. That would be reckless. Instead, I recommend that you take time to understand the risks and benefits of a drug *before* you opt for treatment. You have to make the right choice for yourself and work with your health-care practitioner to come to the best solution. You may need to take certain medications in spite of your plant-based diet, and that is okay.

Your health doesn't have to be dependent on drugs. Rather, you can ease (or avoid) health complications when you commit to a healthy, active lifestyle — including a plant-based diet. And if there are one or two medications you *have* to take, that's okay. Remember, it's your body, not your doctor's or pharmacist's, so it's up to you to decide which drugs to take, if any.

You can find so many wonderful ways to offset the use and effects of drugs. The world of natural medicine, if approached in a balanced way, includes therapies like supplements, homeopathic remedies, acupuncture, chiropractic care, and dietary protocols that are 100 percent plant-based. These methods have been known to reverse the effects of conditions like diabetes and cancer, and people can often stop taking their medications over a period of time (with the guidance of their health-care practitioner, of course).

Staying well naturally, without the use of drugs or even frequent conventional medical care, is not only possible; it may be the most successful strategy you can employ to increase your longevity. If you adhere to a healthy lifestyle, you may not ever need medications in the first place.

Search online for nutritionally oriented physicians who avoid prescribing pharmaceuticals, or ask around to find a physician like this in your area.

Table 20-1 shows a few common medical conditions and potential plant-based treatments.

Table 20-1	Natural treatment alternatives for common ailments
Health condition	**Natural alternative**
High cholesterol	Lose weight, exercise regularly, and eat nutritious and high-fiber plant foods like apples, bananas, carrots, dried beans, garlic, and grapefruit.
Acid reflux	Lose the belly and avoid heavy meals after 6 p.m. Eat alkaline foods like green veggies, fruits, nuts, seeds, and whole grains.
Arthritis	Try daily stretching exercises, pool workouts, and physical therapy. Eat sulfur-containing foods like asparagus, garlic, and onions. Pineapple, flaxseeds, and rice bran are also known to be helpful.
High blood sugar	Engage in regular vigorous exercise and work with a nutritionist to get the weight off. Eat a diet rich in fiber from whole grains, leafy vegetables, and beans.
High blood pressure	Engage in biofeedback (a process in which different instruments give you info on and help you improve your health) or try yoga. Eat foods like apples, bananas, broccoli, cabbage, and squash, along with grains like millet and buckwheat.
Common cold	Have confidence in the knowledge that colds are caused by viruses, and antibiotics kill only bacteria. Consume fresh vitamin C from broccoli, citrus fruits, strawberries, and other green vegetables.

A key reason doctors prescribe so many medications is that (understandably) the vast majority of patients wants a quick fix. I mean, who likes being sick or in pain? However, you can do a lot to help yourself through diet.

Good health requires lifestyle changes and a few dollars spent out of pocket. The truth is, many seniors should meet with a nutritionist or fitness trainer (pssst — you don't have to wait until your golden years to do that!). Sometimes people reject this because their health insurance won't pay for it, but see if you can save up a little so you don't have to allow your insurance company to control your health and ultimately your longevity. Sock some money away so you can access the care you want and need.

Recognizing dangerous interactions between medicines and foods

Healthy eating is critical for patients who are battling long-term diseases. In fact, it can help reverse a condition or reduce the need for medication. But even healthy foods, including fruits and vegetables, can cause unintended and possibly dangerous interactions with certain medications.

Perhaps the best-known example is grapefruit, which, along with pomegranate, can alter the way certain cholesterol medications work. An enzyme in grapefruit juice blocks the wall of the intestine and prevents many drugs, including cholesterol medication, from being absorbed into the body.

Other examples include some leafy green veggies, such as spinach and kale. Their high vitamin-K levels pose risks for patients being treated with blood thinners to prevent strokes. The following foods have also been known anecdotally to interfere with blood thinners; however, the scientific research is inconclusive: avocados, cranberry juice, flaxseeds, garlic, ginger, mangos, papayas, seaweed, and soy.

To minimize your risk, make sure that you keep your health-care professional up to date about the medications and natural products you're taking. This includes vitamins, minerals, and herbal products.

If you're eating a plant-based diet, tell your doctor or pharmacist so he or she can help you avoid interactions like the ones I mention.

Chapter 21

Purely Fit on a Plant-Based Diet

In This Chapter

▶ Learning the benefits of regular exercise

▶ Keeping things flowing with a variety of activity

Studies show that even 15 minutes of exercise a few times a week is beneficial, but ideally you should get 30 minutes of exercise at least four or five times a week, varying between cardiovascular activity and strength training. The most important thing is simply getting started, though, so put on your gym shoes — it's time to get moving!

Of course, trying to achieve a fitness goal on exercise alone is just half the battle. Eating a complementary plant-based diet helps you achieve results much more quickly and helps you feel better overall. A plant-based diet offers so many nutritional benefits for any level of activity.

In this chapter, I address how being active is an asset to overall health and well-being. I also detail how exercise complements your plant-based diet to help you reach your optimum health. Eating a highly nutritious plant-based diet combined with regular exercise is a recipe for amazing health! The benefits are numerous, so let's get into them.

Checking Out the Benefits of Regular Exercise

Being active helps your cardiovascular health, digestion, and skin, and it also gives you happy endorphins to fuel your day with energy, vibrancy, and power. Exercise can become addictive — in a good way!

You don't need an expensive gym membership and the top equipment to get in shape. Your workouts can be as little as 20 minutes a day. Whether you're an elite athlete or a beginner, you can always find room for variety and balance. Just remember: Working out doesn't have to feel like a chore; it should be enjoyable and fun.

Any exercise is better than *no* exercise, and sometimes you have to start out easy. If you currently don't exercise at all, try taking small steps. Begin by taking a 10-minute walk a few times a week. As you become more used to the activity, take longer walks or walk more quickly.

Improves well-being

The effect that exercise has on a person's well-being is almost impossible to describe in words. It's that euphoric feeling you get after you've completed a workout. Of course, the feeling *before* you work out is very different and may be caused by a lack of motivation (in other words, you'd rather eat that chocolate cupcake over there). But after you bite the bullet and take a step in the right direction of exercise, you feel more than rewarded. Exercise can help:

- **Relieve stress and anxiety.** And because stress affects your immune system and increases blood pressure, relieving unnecessary stress should be a top priority for everyone.

- **Slow age-related decline.** Exercise increases your stamina, as well as bone and muscle strength, flexibility, and balance, which all become more important as you age.

- **Fight depression.** Serotonin levels increase with exercise, so risk of depression is reduced.

- **Promote inner peace.** Exercise helps you mentally and emotionally by increasing the love and respect you have for yourself.

Another thing to consider is that taking time to unwind after a long day at work is just as important as your daily workouts. Try meditation or yoga in the mornings or evenings. Yoga can help you create a mental and physical connection with your body.

Your plant-based diet can also promote well-being, which is why in many cultures vegetarianism goes hand in hand with meditation. Also, because plants are easy to digest, a plant-based diet makes it easier to meditate and relax your mind and body.

Builds and improves energy

Did you know that working out gives you more energy? New research suggests that regular exercise can increase energy levels, even among people suffering from chronic medical conditions associated with fatigue, such as cancer and heart disease. Researchers say nearly every group studied — from healthy adults to cancer patients to those with chronic conditions, including diabetes and heart disease — benefited from exercise.

To support your physical activity, plant-based foods provide all the macronutrients (proteins, carbohydrates, and fats) that are essential in maximizing and maintaining the optimal energy you get from working out. Because working out causes physical stress, it creates acidity in the body. Your plant-based diet helps your body neutralize that and regain a state of alkalinity.

Following are some of my favorite plant-based energy-boosting foods. These are the foods I reach for when I want to get moving, and I highly suggest them to anyone who hasn't tried them yet. I know that my body's going to use them efficiently and that they'll give me that boost of energy without causing me to crash and burn. They're sustaining, nourishing, and versatile enough that I can consume them daily in multiple ways without ever getting bored of them.

Go ahead, give these a try:

- ✔ **Hempseeds:** Contain omega-3 fats and provide long-sustaining energy. Put them on salads, in smoothies, and in cereal.

- ✔ **Chia seeds:** Are loaded with fiber and expand when soaked. Chia makes the most delicious morning porridge (see recipes in Chapters 10 and 14). Amazing as pre-workout nutrition.

- ✔ **Kale:** Is a green leafy powerhouse veggie. It's loaded with magnesium and is alkaline forming. Chopped up in a raw salad or steamed on the side with quinoa, kale completes any plate.

- ✔ **Sea vegetables:** Storing a wide range of trace minerals and nutrients, sea vegetables provide natural sodium. My favorite sea vegetables are arame and nori — they give mental clarity and focus. See Chapter 4 for more on sea vegetables.

- ✔ **Tempeh:** It's one of the highest sources of plant protein, is fermented, and is easy to digest. I love marinating tempeh with cider vinegar, lemon juice, and coconut oil for a boost to salads and wraps.

- ✔ **Coconut water and coconut oil:** Coconut water replenishes the body with much-needed electrolytes. So when you're working out, this should be your go-to beverage. Coconut oil is loaded with medium-chain fats, so it's a quick source of energy and nourishment before and after activity.

- ✔ **Quinoa:** Contains all the essential amino acids, which are crucial building blocks for protein. Protein builds muscle, so it's important to consume protein, especially after a workout.

- ✔ **Goji berries:** Are a natural source of antioxidants, protein, and fiber. They're perfect in a trail mix before a workout or great tossed in a smoothie after a workout.

- ✔ **Cacao:** One of nature's richest sources of magnesium. It gives a natural boost of energy, and it's the perfect excuse to have chocolate for breakfast. Tossed in a smoothie or cereal, it adds the perfect crunch and kick.

- ✔ **Honey:** Loaded with enzymes and antibacterial and antimicrobial properties, honey is soothing and easy to take down. It's a natural source of sugar and calories, so it makes a perfect addition to a pre-workout snack, and it also provides an extra boost of energy.

Boosts metabolism

Being active helps boost metabolism by making your muscles work harder, which burns more calories and helps keep your weight in check. You can partake in cardio interval or resistance training, both of which can help you engage your metabolism and achieve a new balance for your body.

Cardio interval training involves short bursts of high-intensity exercise (for example, running, cycling, or any other cardio) for a period of time, followed by a period of rest. You repeat this for between 15 and 30 minutes for an effective metabolism-boosting workout. Additionally, cardio workouts improve circulation and your overall body function.

High-intensity resistance training is all about your body pushing or pulling weight, engaging your muscles directly. This can be in the form of *kettle bell* (a spherical weight with a handle) swings or short, quick reps with a lighter weight or resistance band. This helps get your muscles firing and working quickly to help boost metabolism. In fact, your muscles continue to burn energy (calories) long after you've stopped working out!

Here again your plant-based diet is the perfect partner to your workouts. To really put the turbo in your metabolism boost, consume fruits and vegetables. These have fiber, water, vitamins, and minerals and are amazing sources of antioxidants. Whole grains are also good, as they have a slow release of glucose, some protein, B vitamins, minerals, and fiber. Additionally, legumes and beans contain proteins that are complementary to grain proteins, B vitamins, minerals, fiber, and antioxidants. Nuts and seeds have essential fatty acids, good-quality protein, vitamins, minerals, and cancer-fighting substances, such as fiber. All of these should be included as part of a balanced approach to boosting your metabolism.

Kick it up a notch and enjoy some of these top metabolism-boosting plant-based foods:

- **Grapefruit:** Grapefruit helps "rev" your metabolism by promoting insulin resistance and weight loss. Try enjoying half a grapefruit before meals to reap the effects.

- **Green tea:** It's not the caffeine in green tea that boosts metabolism but rather the antioxidant family called catechins. They have a thermogenic effect that helps promote fat burning. Consider drinking a cup of green tea in the morning a few times a week (or more).

- **Ginger:** Ginger is a stimulant, so it helps boost metabolism and increase energy — especially during exercise. Ginger also helps suppress cortisol (a steroid hormone that is required to regulate energy and mobilization) production, relieve stress, and prevent weight gain.

- **Avocado:** I know you're thinking, "How does this burn fat if it is a fat?" Well, it's important to know that the fats in avocados are polyunsaturated and monounsaturated fats, which help speed up your basal metabolic rate — speeding up your metabolism even when you're sitting down. The fat in avocados is also very satiating and may help curb cravings for other foods.

Enhances immunity

Regular physical activity can help your immune system fight off simple bacterial and viral infections. In addition, having a stronger immune system can decrease your chances of developing other health problems, such as heart disease, osteoporosis, and cancer. Here are a few theories about why:

- Physical activity may help by flushing bacteria from the lungs (preventing colds and flu) and by increasing the body's output of waste, such as urine and sweat.

- Exercise helps antibodies (white blood cells) move around the body more rapidly. In this way, they can detect illnesses earlier than usual. Our body is smart, and these cells somehow have a way of "warning" other cells of intruding bacteria or viruses. Amazing!

- The temporary rise in body temperature during exercise may prevent bacterial growth, allowing the body to fight infection more effectively (similar to when you have a fever).

- Exercise slows down the release of stress-related hormones. Stress can increase the chance of illness.

Get some sleep to feel better

Sleep is a time for the body to repair all the damage that occurs during the day. It's an important part of cleaning up toxins, removing waste, and letting the immune system get to work, and it helps us let go of a lot of the physical, emotional, and mental baggage we accumulate all day.

As several studies report, people who get at least six to seven hours of sleep aren't as susceptible to contracting disease, have a greater ability to focus, and are less prone to developing depression than those who sleep less. Lack of sleep can cause your brain function to sharply decline, making it hard to reason and make decisions. Without proper sleep, our bodies can't repair the previous day's cellular wear and tear.

But you also don't want to get too much sleep, which can be a depressor. Six to seven hours of sleep is adequate for most adults. Set your alarm on your days off, unless your natural body alarm works just fine. (The more regular your sleep cycles are, the more your body remembers when you're tired and when to wake you up.)

It's not just about quantity, though; we need better *quality* sleep (in the deep delta phase). This phase is when growth hormone is released, naturally triggering cellular repair and regeneration. Delta-phase sleep is possible only when one's cortisol level is low. A healthy plant-based diet improves cortisol levels and thus the quality of sleep.

For most people, the best sleep happens between 10 p.m. and 5 a.m. This is when your body does most of its repair and regeneration, allowing you to not only wake up refreshed but also perform at your best during the day.

Although exercise is beneficial, be careful not to overdo it. People who exercise regularly or train hard are at higher risk for overtraining. It can be counterproductive because it decreases the amount of white blood cells in the body and increases the presence of stress-related hormones, leading to sickness and overall malaise.

Plant-based foods play a role in immunity-boosting, too. They're anti-inflammatory, rich in antioxidants, rich in phytonutrients, and nutrient-dense, and they provide an array of minerals and vitamins. They also offer additional benefits, such as help in maintaining healthy cholesterol, blood pressure, and body weight. They help you maintain the ideal pH balance and aid in a natural detoxification process, and most importantly they're tasty and flavorful and have no additives or chemicals. (Flip to Chapter 23 to read about ten foods that can help you boost your immunity.)

Prevents illness

Exercise has a profound effect on the prevention and treatment of chronic diseases, such as heart disease, cancer, and diabetes. Exercise can help offset diseases by helping promote lymph movement through the body, removing waste, and releasing hormones that have a positive effect on all systems of the body. It helps with circulation and overall cardio, moving fat deposits in the body and keeping weight maintained, thereby stabilizing blood-sugar levels.

On top of regular exercise, living on a plant-based diet reduces your risk of oxidative stress and chronic inflammation, which are big culprits in many chronic illnesses. Some experts believe that chronic inflammation of the brain from excessive oxidative stress is the major cause of the symptoms and behaviors seen in attention-deficit disorder and Alzheimer's disease. Excessive oxidative stress can be triggered by gluten intolerance or sensitivity caused by a leaky gut. Other causes include casein (a dairy-based protein), food allergies and sensitivities, inadequate antioxidant intake, and excessive animal-protein intake.

Don't Think, Just Move

The key to getting started is to just start. Find something to do and get your body moving. The longer you spend thinking about what activity you should take up, the more time you're missing out on getting that body moving. It's okay if you don't know whether you like something; try it anyway! The only way to know whether you like it is to give it a go. If you find you don't like it, move on to the next type of exercise. Keep trying until you find something that gels with you. The following sections offer some types of exercise you may want to try.

If you're looking to get into some activity but aren't sure how much to do, how often to do it, or which activity is right for you, seek the advice of your health-care professional or a fitness specialist. This is especially important if you're beyond a certain age or have been diagnosed with conditions that can be aggravated by physical activity. It's always best to ask first, just in case. The goal is to have fun, feel good, and get results.

Cross-training

Many people enjoy walking or running because it's such an easy way to exercise.

High-impact exercise like this is crucial, but it raises the risk of injury during training, especially if this is your *only* form of activity. Cross-training can help you prevent injury from repetitive motion or heavy impact. Simply spend time doing an activity that works different muscles and involves different motions. Changing things up day to day or week to week is one of the best ways to challenge your body while staying safe and injury free.

Four popular cross-training modes are cycling, swimming, elliptical exercise, and stepping. All are low- or non-impact exercises that provide excellent aerobic workouts. That makes all of these valuable training options, especially for runners. The elliptical trainer and the stepper in particular are good substitutes for running when running isn't possible — when you're injured, for example. But apart from reducing the volume of impact, working on these machines won't add anything to your running that running itself doesn't provide. Of those four cross-training options, only one effectively works muscle groups that are complementary to running: cycling.

If walking, running, or cycling isn't your thing, consider joining a gym and trying out some fun cross-fit classes. Or pick up a copy of *Cross-Training For Dummies* by Tony Ryan and Martica Heaner (Wiley) and try out the exercises on your own.

Resistance

Strength resistance training is beneficial for so many reasons. In addition to building muscle, it can help burn more calories, build up bone strength and health, and get your blood flowing.

Here are some of the top ways to get started:

- ✔ Kettle-bell training
- ✔ Resistance band
- ✔ Medicine ball
- ✔ Free weights
- ✔ Body-weight squats and lunges
- ✔ Push-ups
- ✔ Sit-ups
- ✔ Planks and side planks
- ✔ Gym equipment/machines

If you're interested in these kinds of exercises, check out *Weight Training For Dummies* by Liz Neporent, Suzanne Schlosberg, and Shirley J. Archer (Wiley).

Floor work (yoga, Pilates, stretching)

Floor work is a blanket term for full-body exercise and conditioning methods that work your body head to toe. Some examples include yoga, Pilates, and general stretching. Floor work has many fantastic benefits, beyond toning and stretching, that many people aren't familiar with.

One of the biggest benefits is the relaxation component — it makes you feel so uplifted after finishing a workout! Also, because you have a complete mind-body connection the whole time, your thoughts or worries often release as you direct your focus to the movement. If you're prone to stress, this is a great way of centering yourself by focusing on breath and movement.

When you have this mind-body connection, your body awareness increases, which is extremely beneficial if you play sports, want to have a better understanding of your body, or always seem to be stiff and sore and wonder why.

Benefits of working out at home

Going to the gym can be tedious. You have to get dressed, drive to the gym, and change into your workout clothes. Then, after working out, you have to do it all again in the opposite order. All of this can take more time than the actual workout. Add to this the fact that gym membership costs are more and more expensive because of the amount of activities offered. If you're not a fan of the gym, why not try working out at home?

At the top of the list of benefits is that working out at home gives you flexibility. You can work out in the morning, in the evening, or on alternate mornings and evenings to make the best use of your time.

And although gyms certainly have a more social quality than your home can offer, being social doesn't make your workout effective. Often, the opposite is true. Many gym members aren't really there to work out. They go to pass some time and meet people. Sometimes, gym patrons even think it's strange to see people who are seriously working out.

And finally, there's a real joy and relaxation that comes from knowing that no one will disturb you while you're exercising to discuss the weather or tell you that you're not exercising the right way (this is especially a great perk if you feel shy or self-conscious). At home, you can remain focused and have a faster, more productive workout (provided you first hide all the distractions, such as your phone and computer — unless you're using them to watch exercise or yoga videos!).

Try these things at home:

- ✔ Resistance exercises: If you don't have weights or an exercise band, feel free to get creative. Use things you find around the house, such as five-pound bags of flour, buckets of water, or even small children!

- ✔ Cardio training: Maybe you've invested in a treadmill or elliptical trainer at home. If so, dust it off and put it to use.

- ✔ Workout DVDs or videos, which may include anything from body-weight exercises to yoga or Pilates.

- ✔ Jumping rope.

- ✔ Calisthenics, such as jumping jacks, push-ups, sit-ups, or jogging in place.

- ✔ Rebounder or trampoline exercise.

- ✔ Workout programs on home gaming systems: You can do just about anything, including full-body workouts that track your movements and increase the challenge over time. Technology is amazing!

An added bonus of this type of workout is that you can do it solo in your home or an outdoor setting that you find serene, or you can join a class if you like being part of a group.

If you want a taste of these different types of floor exercises, grab a copy of *Stretching For Dummies* by LaReine Chabut with Madeleine Lewis, *Yoga For Dummies* by Georg Feuerstein and Larry Payne, or *Pilates For Dummies* by Ellie Herman. All are published by Wiley.

Team sports

Doing things solo may not be your thing, so join a team! You may be one of those people who grew up playing hockey, baseball, or football, which is great. As a regular part of your routine, playing team sports has all kinds of benefits (not just the high physical activity level, which is a huge perk, of course). Team sports give you a chance to socialize, work together, and build each other up. Of course, the other nice thing is that everyone shares a commitment to show up. You have other people keeping you accountable and expecting you to be there, so the exercise is more meaningful, and it's more likely that you'll stick with your activity. It also means you have something to look forward to on a regular basis, whether that's every week or every month.

Here are some of the most common team sports to try out:

- ✔ Tennis
- ✔ Baseball or softball
- ✔ Hockey
- ✔ Football
- ✔ Volleyball
- ✔ Basketball
- ✔ Soccer

Want to find a recreational team or league to join? Try doing a search on Meetup.com or other social media and check out your local parks and recreation department or YMCA.

As a plant-based eater on a team, you may notice that you're one of only a few, as most people don't eat a very healthy diet even when playing sports. Also, you'll usually face the misconception that you need meat and milk to stay strong and play harder and better. Well, this is where you can be the one to introduce healthy snacks and drink options (as I note in Chapter 19) for fueling up before, during, and after the game.

Part V
The Part of Tens

the part of tens

For a list of ten kid-friendly plant-based meals, head to www.dummies.com/extras/plantbaseddiet.

In this part . . .

- Identify ten tricky foods that aren't plant-based.

- Explore how you can boost your immune system with super-nutritious plant-based foods.

- Discover plant-based foods to use for skin and beauty treatments.

- See why eating meat is bad for you, for animals, and for the planet.

Chapter 22

Ten Foods That Are Surprisingly Not Plant-Based

Don't be fooled — some non-plant-based foods present themselves as plant-based. Look closely at labels on these innocent-looking foods, and you may find ingredients you don't want in your body. Some of the foods you think are safe actually aren't. This chapter gives you a rundown of some common foods that may be fooling you.

Bread

This supermarket aisle is usually a disappointment for us plant-based eaters. Many well-known national brands use non-plant-based ingredients. Many whole-wheat breads contain milk products, for example, and some traditional Italian breads contain lard. But better supermarkets also stock bread from a local bakery. You have to check the ingredients, but locally baked bread is frequently vegan. Oddly, these local breads are often kept in a different aisle than the national brands.

The solution? Look for breads that are made from 100 percent whole grains and have either active cultures (for sourdough bread) or other added ingredients like nuts, seeds, or even legumes. You should be able to recognize every ingredient in your bread. If you're savvy in the kitchen, make your own bread instead.

Don't confuse locally baked breads with ones from the supermarket's in-house bakery, which typically bakes some of the most compromising bread ever produced. Check the ingredients and you'll see what I'm talking about.

Soup Stock Powders or Cartons

If you're making soup at home, you may be looking for a great base or stock to get it going. Be wary of some of the seemingly vegetarian stocks or even "mock" chicken stocks on your store's shelves, because these items may contain traces of animal fat or other animal products.

The solution? Make your own stocks from leftover veggie scraps, sea vegetables, or even herbs sprinkled in water. This is the cleanest way to enjoy a broth, and you know exactly what's going into it! One of my favorite broths involves adding a piece of kombu (seaweed) to water and then building my soup from there. Check out Chapter 11 for advice on making soups and some yummy soup recipes.

If you'd rather not make your own soup stock, look for packages that state "no animal-derived ingredients."

Veggie Burgers or Sausages

It's funny to think that a "veggie" burger may have non-plant-based ingredients in it. That's why you have to be extremely vigilant about reading labels. Many brands contain trace amounts of milk or eggs.

The solution? Be sure to look for brands that are made exclusively from organic soy (and not isolated soy protein, which is extremely processed), tempeh, whole grains, or nuts and seeds, with just veggies and herbs added. The next phase, of course, is to make your own veggie burgers and sausages. Try out some of the recipes in this book (see Chapter 12 for a great one)!

Worcestershire Sauce

Worcestershire sauce contains anchovies, which are certainly not suitable for plant-based eaters.

The solution? Grab a bottle of tamari (fermented soy sauce). Tamari is completely vegan and can be used in place of Worcestershire sauce, both in recipes and as a condiment.

Alcoholic Beverages

The one item that I'm sure you don't want to know contains non-plant-based ingredients is alcohol. Unfortunately, most filtering practices use some kind of animal product, particularly in the production of beers, wines, and ciders.

The solution? Vegan wines do exist! Of course, when you buy one, you're probably getting a beverage that's also organic or local (and will therefore likely taste better). Do some exploring and try something new. You can usually find alternatives at your local liquor store, bar, or winery. Just ask.

Noodles and Pasta

Many noodles in restaurants and stores are made with eggs, which is fair, because traditional pasta includes eggs as part of the recipe.

The solution? Most dried pasta varieties that are whole-grain and gluten-free are suitable for plant-based eaters, because they're made with just the whole grain and water. If you're dining out, ask your server about the pasta to make sure it's egg-free (flip to Chapter 16 for more ideas about how to navigate restaurant dining).

Dairy-Free Cheese

Although you may assume that soy-, nut-, and rice-based "cheeses" are non-dairy, they often contain some form of casein or whey protein.

The solution? To be safe, look for products labeled "vegan," which indicates that they are, in fact, dairy-free. Be sure to read all the ingredients, searching for words like *rennet*, *evaporated milk powder*, or *casein*. You can also try making your own dairy-free cheeses from cashews. Nutritional yeast is also a great solution, along with avocado. See Chapter 7 for a list of alternatives to this favorite comfort food.

Granola

Granola is traditionally prepared with a mixture of raw grains, dried fruits, nuts, and seeds that are tossed with a sweetener and either butter or oil. Although there's no rule of thumb about which granolas use which fats, it's often the case that oil-based granola will be labeled as such. However, if you're at a buffet, resort, or restaurant, there's no way of knowing from where the granola is sourced or with what it's made if it's not made in-house.

The solution? Luckily, granola is incredibly easy to prepare and makes your home smell wonderful as it bakes. Try out my dairy-free granola recipe in Chapter 10 and see for yourself.

Coconut oil is my substitute for butter in most baked goods. Oils such as grapeseed can be used, too (more on oils in Chapter 12).

Boxed Cereal and Cereal Bars

More boxed cereals than you'd ever suspect contain some form of dairy, even "health food" and "natural" cereals. Usually they contain casein, nonfat milk powder, whey protein, or whey protein isolates.

Aside from the obvious "yogurt" varieties, many cereal bars contain some form of dairy — typically butter fat, casein, milk powder, or whey.

The solution? Many varieties of cereal are now made from whole grains with no added traces of dairy. Look for brands that are relatively plain so you can upgrade them yourself at home with rice milk, almond milk, and other toppings, such as coconut and fruit. Making oatmeal from scratch is another safe solution to make sure your breakfast is clean and plant-based.

Orange Juice

Orange juice that is enriched with omega-3 fatty acids can have traces of fish oils. Not something you expected to hear, right? Most omega-3-enriched drinks or foods, such as margarine, olive oil, and bread, also may contain fish-based rather than plant-based sources of omega-3 fatty acids.

The solution? Don't buy boxed juices. Instead, make your own fresh-pressed juices or, if you must buy premade juice, look for juices that are 100 percent from fruit sources and not enriched with other nutrients.

Chapter 23

Ten Plant-Based Foods That Boost Your Immunity

In This Chapter

▷ Adding potent whole foods into your diet

▷ Kicking a cold with cayenne pepper

▷ Making healing teas

▷ Trying the plant-based alternative to chicken-noodle soup

*T*he plant world contains a natural army of foods that are ready to fight — infections, that is! Getting a steady supply of the following foods helps you build up immunity so that, when that cold comes for you, you may be able to block it entirely — or, at the very least, not let it affect you as much. In addition to eating these ten foods regularly, you can use them to make home remedies at the first sign of a cold or flu!

Garlic

The most pungent of the plant kingdom inhabitants (well, at least to me), garlic contains the immune-stimulating compound allicin, which promotes the activity of white blood cells to destroy cold and flu viruses. It also stimulates other immune cells, which fight viral, fungal, and bacterial infections. Garlic kills with near 100 percent effectiveness the human rhinovirus, which causes colds, common flu, and respiratory viruses.

Because allicin is released when you cut, chop, chew, or crush *raw* cloves, allow freshly chopped garlic to stand for 10 minutes and then cook it, sprinkle it over foods, drop it into soup, or swallow bits of garlic with some water like a pill. You can also drop a clove of garlic into some honey and swallow it immediately for a quick dose that tastes good!

Did you know that most detoxing happens through your feet at night? To take advantage of this, and because garlic *loves* to fight bacteria and infections, some people crush garlic in olive oil to make a paste and rub it on their feet. They then put socks on and let the garlic do its work while they sleep.

Onions

Onions, like garlic, contain allicin. They also contain quercetin, a nutrient that breaks up mucus in your head and chest while boosting your immune system. Additionally, the pungency of onions increases your blood circulation and makes you sweat, which is helpful during cold weather to help prevent infections. Consuming raw onion within a few hours of the first symptoms of a cold or flu produces a strong immune effect.

 Chopping onions into your favorite soup or cooked recipe is a great way to enjoy them. Also, it may sound a little weird, but putting half an onion in your bedroom while you sleep can help absorb some of the circulating bacteria and potentially lessen the symptoms of your cold.

Ginger

Spicy, pungent, and delicious, ginger reduces fevers, soothes sore throats, and encourages coughing to remove mucus from the chest. Anti-inflammatory chemicals like shagaol and gingerol give ginger that spicy kick that stimulates blood circulation and opens your sinuses. Improved circulation means more oxygen is getting to your tissues to help remove toxins and viruses. Research has indicated that ginger can help prevent and treat the flu. Ginger is also extremely helpful for stomachaches, nausea, and headaches.

 If you're feeling a little sickly, a homemade ginger tea is one of the best things you can drink. Slice some fresh ginger root, place it into a pot with water, and bring to a boil. Then drop in a bit of lemon juice or cayenne, which makes the tea that much more effective at nourishing and purifying your system.

Cayenne

The cayenne family of hot peppers (cayenne, habanero, Scotch bonnet, and bird peppers, to name a few) contains capsicum — a rich source of vitamin C and bioflavonoids, which aid your immune system in fighting colds and flus. It does this by increasing the production of white blood cells, which cleanse your cells and tissues of toxins. Cayenne pepper is also full of beta carotene and antioxidants that support your immune system and help build healthy mucus membrane tissue that defends against viruses and bacteria. Spicy cayenne peppers raise your body's temperature to make you sweat, increasing the activity of your immune system.

You can use cayenne that is found in the spice aisle; however, the ground cayenne isn't as potent as a fresh pepper. The fresher the pepper, the more effective it is. However, fresher also means spicier, so choose accordingly.

When you're sick, add organic cayenne powder to some warm water with lemon juice for an intense immune boost.

Squash

Squash is a good source of vitamin C and carotene. The six carotenoids (out of the 600 found in nature) found most commonly in human tissue — and supplied by squash and other gourds — decrease the risk of various cancers, protect the eyes and skin from the effects of ultraviolet light, and defend against heart disease. One of them, alpha-carotene, helps slow down the aging process. Butternut squash is the strongest source of these nutrients, but you can also try acorn, Hubbard, delicata, calabaza, and spaghetti squash.

Whether roasted in the oven or pureed into a soup, butternut squash is sweet and delicious and will warm your body from the inside out! Any of the items in this chapter can be combined to make a delicious squash soup on days you're feeling less than 100 percent.

Kale

Like other leafy greens, kale offers up a good dose of vitamin E. This immunity-boosting antioxidant is known for increasing the production of B cells, those white blood cells that kill unwanted bacteria. Whether you eat kale raw in a salad, steam it, or lightly sauté it, you'll reap all of its wonderful benefits.

Citrus Fruits

Adding a bit of citrus to your diet goes a long way toward fending off your next cold or flu. Packed with vitamin C, oranges and grapefruits help increase your body's resistance to nasty invaders.

The best way to enjoy citrus fruits is to eat them whole. Otherwise, you can make fresh juice yourself (stay away from the premade stuff in cartons or in the freezer section at your supermarket). You can also squeeze some fresh lemon juice into some water, either warm or at room temperature, for a healing beverage. Lemon juice is pretty sour, so add it gradually to avoid making an undrinkable beverage.

Green Tea

Green tea is a potent source of antioxidants called polyphenols — especially catechins. Some studies have found that catechins can destroy the influenza and common cold viruses.

Sipping a hot cup of green tea when you're feeling under the weather can really help you come alive again. Try adding some honey or lemon to kick it up a bit.

Miso Soup

Miso soup is the plant-based version of chicken-noodle soup. It has wonderful healing properties that are amazing at boosting immunity. As a living food, miso is loaded with enzymes and healthy bacteria that help fight infection and keep your cells thriving.

All you need is one teaspoon of miso paste stirred into a mug or bowl of warm water, and you're set. Sip this down, especially at the first sign of a cold or when you're just feeling "off" with a stomachache, headache, or something like that. This is sure to hit the spot and make you feel good all over.

Mushrooms

For centuries, people around the world have turned to mushrooms for a healthy immune system. Contemporary researchers now know why. Studies show that mushrooms increase the production and activity of white blood cells, making them more aggressive. This is a good thing when you have an infection.

Shiitake, maitake, chaga, and reishi mushrooms appear to pack the biggest immunity punch. Experts recommend eating a quarter ounce to an ounce a few times a day for maximum immune benefits. If you're sick, having mushrooms in tea form or as an extract is the best way to go for immediate results.

Chapter 24

Ten Plant-Based Beauty Treatments to Use on Your Skin

In This Chapter

▷ Using plant-based foods to moisturize

▷ Discovering how to make homemade masks out of your favorite fruits

▷ Understanding the power of lemon juice

Did you know that any good commercial beauty product likely contains extracts of plant-based whole foods? If you look at the ingredients closely, you'll see them — maybe hidden between all the other (toxic) chemicals that are put into most skin products. My question to you is, why not go right to the source and put these foods directly on your skin, without the fillers and additives? This approach not only saves you money but also saves your skin (*plus*, if you happen to get some in your mouth, it can be downright delicious!).

Avocado

Using avocado is an excellent, natural way to nourish and care for your body without any abrasive chemicals. Essential and extra-virgin avocado oil has long been used in beauty products such as hair conditioners, moisturizers, cleansers, and facials. This is because avocado is a rich source of several essential nutrients that refresh and moisturize your skin.

Avocados are among the healthiest natural ingredients on the planet. They contain more than 25 vital nutrients, including A, B, C, E, and K vitamins and minerals such as copper, potassium, iron, magnesium, and phosphorus. Additionally:

✔ The vitamin A in avocados helps with purging dead skin cells.

✔ The glutamine amino acid present in avocados cleanses your skin and offers it protection against harsh environmental factors.

✔ The antioxidants in avocados detoxify your body by removing toxins that tend to cause premature aging of the skin. They also help eliminate wrinkles, giving your skin a youthful glow.

Scoop out the flesh of a ripe avocado, mash it in a bowl, and smear it on your skin for a nourishing mask. Leave it on for at least 20 minutes before washing it off.

Coconut

Coconut oil, which you can buy in glass bottles, makes a great moisturizer from head to toe, particularly for dry lips and rough hands and feet. You can even use it on your scalp and for your hair.

Coconut oil and coconut cream have been used as food and medicine since the dawn of history. Ayurveda (the traditional medicine of India) and the traditional medicinal systems of Polynesia have long advocated the coconut's therapeutic and cosmetic properties.

Raw Honey

Bee products are considered to be among the most spiritual and magical foods on the planet. Honey in its organic (wild), raw, and unfiltered state is rich in minerals, antioxidants, probiotics, and enzymes. Honey is an extremely healing food that provides the body with a digestible and soothing form of sugar (energy).

Raw honey is also incredible for your skin, thanks to its antibacterial properties and hefty serving of skin-saving antioxidants. Whether you're looking for an inexpensive DIY solution or a powerful skin treatment, raw honey can help you regain your glow. Here's a rundown of its benefits:

- ✔ Honey is naturally antibacterial, so it's great for acne treatment and prevention.
- ✔ Full of antioxidants, it's great for slowing down aging.
- ✔ It's extremely moisturizing and soothing, so it helps create a glow.
- ✔ Honey is clarifying because it opens up pores, making them easy to unclog.

The best way to use honey is to apply it topically as is (undiluted). That way, your skin can soak up all of its goodness. After about 15 minutes, rinse it off. You may need two rinses to get it all off!

Raw honey and pasteurized honey are very different. Basically, *don't* buy honey if it's in a little plastic bear bottle. True honey should actually be unpasteurized and raw. Raw honey sometimes comes as a liquid, but the best form is solid and opaque, and you can typically find it at health or organic food stores. Because honey is a living food, pasteurization kills all the enzymes and beneficial nutrients present in raw honey. So be sure to look for a label that says "raw" or "unpasteurized." Bonus: It also tastes better!

Lemon Juice

Fresh lemon juice is loaded with healthy vitamins, so it's useful both as a food and as a home remedy for many disorders. A lesser-known fact, however, is that lemon juice also has many benefits when applied directly to the skin.

The acids in lemon juice may be irritating to some people, so be sure to dilute lemon juice with water before applying it to your skin.

Try using lemon juice in the following ways:

- ✔ Diminish the discoloration caused by scars, certain skin disorders, and age spots by applying lemon juice to the discolored area. It may be helpful to apply the lemon juice at bedtime and leave it on the skin overnight.

- ✔ Use lemon juice on acne and blackheads to reduce the frequency and severity. If you leave lemon juice on the acne and blackheads overnight, be sure to wash it off in the morning.

- ✔ Try lemon juice as a natural exfoliant; the citric acid acts as a gentle "skin peel" that removes the top layer of dead skin cells. This results in a smooth complexion when used regularly. It also helps brighten or lighten the skin, moisturizes and tones, and fights wrinkles.

Apple-Cider Vinegar

Apple-cider vinegar is often recommended as a treatment for age spots and warts and as a hair conditioner, and it helps balance the pH of your skin and hair.

For age spots, use a mixture of one part vinegar to two parts water as a toner. You can also apply undiluted apple-cider vinegar directly to the spots. Preferably, you should do this several times a day for at least a month. Some people have even better results mixing the vinegar with either fresh orange juice or onion juice and applying it several times a day.

Make sure you're applying the mixture to the age spots *only*, perhaps with a cotton ball, as it's likely to sting sensitive skin.

You can treat warts with apple-cider vinegar in a different way. Soak a small cotton ball in the vinegar and use tape or a bandage to keep the soaked cotton ball in contact with the wart for as long as possible. You can either do it in the morning and keep it on all day or do it before bed and wear it overnight. For even faster results, keep it on around the clock, with a change of application each evening. Many people report that this treatment clears up warts in a week. Be aware that the warts may turn black before falling off. Continue with the treatment for a further week, even if the wart looks to be gone, to make sure it doesn't return.

Finally, this may sound strange, but try doing a rinse of apple-cider vinegar after you shampoo instead of using conditioner. It makes your hair lustrous and soft without any harsh chemicals.

Strawberries

Did you know you can put strawberries directly on your face by mushing them into a mask or rubbing them over your skin? They combat oil, work as an antioxidant, and brighten your face. They're also rich in vitamin C, which has amazing benefits for brightening and nourishing your skin. They're also known to whiten your teeth!

Bananas

Bananas whose skins have a few brown spots are perfect for a face mask. This means your bananas are slightly soft and ripe. Bananas exfoliate like crazy and give new life to a dull complexion. They also moisturize and are great for all types of skin. Mush it up (add a little honey if you'd like) and rub it on your face. Leave on for 10 minutes and rinse.

Almonds and Oats

Toss either almonds or whole oats into the food processor and turn them into a powder. Then you can add water and use them as a facial scrub. They moisturize, exfoliate, and cleanse. Almonds are also rich in vitamin E, which has nourishing properties to soothe skin and promote wound-healing.

Instead of water, add some non-dairy milk and turn these scrubs into a luxurious way to soothe dry or sunburned skin. Rub gently on the skin, being careful not to be too abrasive.

Olive Oil

Olive oil is a centuries-old beauty staple. Moisturize your face with it, condition your hair with it, or add some salt to make the easiest hand scrub ever.

A good rule of thumb when buying olive oils (or any oils, really): Go for extra virgin, expeller pressed, and organic when you can. They're higher in antioxidants, contain fewer chemicals, and aren't as "messed with" as more-processed kinds.

Aloe Vera

Aloe vera is a great plant food! It's one of the most nourishing plants on the planet for the skin. Here's why:

- ✔ It's an excellent moisturizer for the skin and helps to rejuvenate, hydrate, and keep your skin looking fresh.
- ✔ Aloe vera has antimicrobial properties, making it ideal to treat acne.
- ✔ It's an amazing natural antioxidant.
- ✔ It's helpful in retaining skin's firmness, making it a great anti-aging skin cream.
- ✔ Aloe vera gel or meat, from the whole leaf, is also known to reduce pain and inflammation both internally and externally. It's most helpful with sunburns, insect bites, rashes, eczema, and cuts and wounds.

Get an aloe vera plant at your local market or garden center. It's not only exotic looking to place in your window at home, but you also have a natural remedy for all your beauty needs all the time! Just pull off a leaf and cut it open, extract the gel, and moisturize away!

Did you know you can scoop out the flesh of aloe vera and put it into your favorite smoothie? It's extremely healing and soothing to the gut and makes your smoothie deliciously creamy!

Chapter 25

Ten Bad Things about Eating Meat

* *

In This Chapter

▶ Realizing the impact that eating animals has on the environment

▶ Understanding how meat can contribute to heart disease, osteoporosis, and cancer

▶ Discovering how factory farming affects the lives of animals

* *

*T*here is no doubt that eating meat creates health concerns not only for consumers but also for the environment and (of course) the farmed animals, and it's unfortunate that people overlook so many of these problems. Animals are taken advantage of, our environment suffers, and ultimately we suffer, as well. Throughout this book I explain why eating plants is the way to go, but in this chapter I explicitly outline the negatives of eating meat.

Meat Production Wastes Natural Resources

The world is a diverse place that offers many natural resources. Sadly, we tend to take advantage of these resources without any real concern for how our use impacts their abundance. The meat industry is one of the ugliest examples of this. It places extreme stress on our natural resources, causing extreme reduction and depletion:

✔ **Water:** The amount of water required to produce a pound of meat is rather disturbing. It takes more than 2,400 gallons of water to produce one pound of meat, whereas it takes only 25 gallons of water to produce one pound of wheat. Additionally, toxins, pesticides, and other residues from the extreme amount of animal waste produced by meat farms end up in nearby water supplies and cause pollution.

✔ **Land:** According to the United Nations, raising animals for food now uses almost 30 percent of our land mass (including land used for grazing and land used to grow feed crops). More than 260 million acres of U.S. forests have been cleared to grow grain to feed farmed animals, and every minute more land is cleared to produce more feedlots.

Additionally, livestock grazing is the number one reason that plant species in North America become threatened and go extinct, and it also leads to soil erosion and barren land. Finally, cattle raising is a primary factor in the destruction of the world's remaining tropical rainforests.

✓ **Food:** Raising animals for food is extremely inefficient. Animals eat large quantities of grain, soybeans, oats, and corn, but they produce comparatively small amounts of meat, dairy products, or eggs in return. More than 70 percent of the grain and cereals we grow in this country are fed to farmed animals. It takes up to 13 pounds of grain to produce just 1 pound of meat, and even fish on fish farms must be fed up to 5 pounds of wild-caught fish to produce 1 pound of farmed fish flesh. Imagine the impact on world hunger if we ate the plants directly. We'd have 13 times more food available to feed people.

✓ **Energy:** Raising animals for food scoops up precious energy. It takes more than 11 times as much fossil fuel to make one calorie from animal protein as it does to make one calorie from plant protein. To get a feel for this, all you need to do is add up the energy-intensive stages of raising animals for food:

1. Grow massive amounts of corn, grain, and soybeans (with all the required tilling, irrigation, crop dusting, and so on).

2. Transport the grain and soybeans to feed manufacturers on gas-guzzling 18-wheelers.

3. Operate the feed mills (requiring massive energy expenditures).

4. Transport the feed to the factory farms (again, in gas-guzzling vehicles).

5. Operate the factory farms.

6. Truck the animals many miles to slaughter.

7. Operate the slaughterhouses.

8. Transport the meat to processing plants.

9. Operate the meat-processing plants.

10. Transport the meat to grocery stores.

11. Keep the meat refrigerated or frozen in the stores until it's sold.

Meat Isn't as Rich in Nutrients as Plants

An animal-based diet isn't as diverse in terms of nutrients as a plant-based diet is. You pretty much get two main macronutrients — protein and fat — with essentially no vitamins or minerals, and no fiber. What most people don't know is that the body needs vitamins and minerals to digest and assimilate protein efficiently. We also need fiber to help the body push things through so we can assimilate nutrients.

Meat intake can build up in the body and slow things down, causing you to feel tired and undernourished. Going plant-based ensures that your body at least gets the nutritional baseline it requires to thrive on a day-to-day basis. For example, eating kale instead of meat provides your body with protein, fiber, vitamins, and minerals, while also giving you energy without weighing you down with excess fat or calories.

Animals Are Fed Poor-Quality Feed

Most conventionally raised animals are fed bottom-of-the-barrel feed that isn't in any way natural to them. This not only leaves animals unsatisfied on many levels but also affects their biological makeup. Many are starved of the nutrients they require to be healthy because they're fed an unnatural diet. This affects not only *their* well-being but ultimately the well-being of meat consumers. The foods these animals eat aren't part of their native diet.

Here are some of the top things animals are fed but should not be eating:

- Parts from other animals (even within their own species)
- High-grain diets, including genetically modified corn and soy (even though most animals are meant to eat grass)
- Unnatural feed (garbage and human leftovers)

In the United States, up to 70 percent of antibiotics are fed to farm animals that aren't even sick. This injudicious use of antibiotics presents a serious and growing threat to human health because the practice creates new strains of dangerous antibiotic-resistant bacteria.

If these animals were living in the wild, they would be eating a diet that contributed to a more natural life and composition of their genetics. But unfortunately, their diets are manipulated by humans, to whom they're merely a commodity. This food, in turn, goes into your body when you consume their meat. *They* get trashy feed, *you* get trashy feed.

If you're in the midst of transitioning or choosing to keep meat as part of your diet, please make plants the priority on your plate and choose wild, organic, or naturally raised meat, poultry, eggs, and fish. A happy animal means a happy you — and it all makes a difference.

One option is to look for products that are "certified humane" by Humane Farm Animal Care. Visit `www.certifiedhumane.org` for more information.

Meat Is Acidic

Meat is one of the major acidic foods in the standard North American diet. It's difficult for the body to break down and digest and requires extra work from the kidneys. As a result, it produces too much acid in the body. Too much acid not only weakens the body's immune defenses, which increases risks for infections, but also contributes to chronic diseases.

The other consideration to look at is the *quality* of meat that a majority of people eat: often it's fried, overcooked, and not eaten alongside green vegetables. This not only creates acidity in the body but also does nothing to help neutralize it. Choosing to eat more plants throughout the day can help balance this ratio.

Meat Is Loaded with Toxins

Animals are sponges that soak up toxicity. Because a majority of their biological makeup is fat, their bodies can accumulate an excessive amount of toxins. So, when the animals eat a toxic diet, these toxins get carried with them for life, and they end up in the food you eat.

For example, livestock can ingest toxins such as pesticides from the conventional produce they eat (that is, of course, if they're not raised organically). Because the cost of organic produce is so much higher, a majority of farmers choose to save money when it comes to animal feed.

Finally, the sea life that swims in our polluted oceans and waterways has incredibly absorbent skin and fat, which is why fish and other seafood are often tainted with mercury and other heavy metals.

Meat Is High in Saturated Fat

It's one of the things we hear a lot these days: "Be mindful of the amount of saturated fat you eat!" Unfortunately, many people get confused about the sources of this unhealthy fat and don't realize that a majority of it is from animals. Saturated fat is healthy for the living animal, but the human body can't break it down in a way that is healthy.

Eating the amount of saturated fat from animals that most people do can lead to major health problems. Additionally, many people are eating fried meats, fatty cuts, and skin, with no care for leaner options — all of which contribute to plaque buildup, heart disease, and other diseases, such as obesity and diabetes.

Eating Meat Can Increase Your Risk for Cancer and Osteoporosis

In addition to causing heart disease, excess meat consumption leads to other health-degrading conditions, such as osteoporosis and even cancer. The excess protein — despite what people may think — isn't good for the body. Also, the accumulation of meat can lead to more fatty deposits in the body, which become plaque deposits, and they can start to calcify and affect many of our tissues and bones, causing long-term diseases like heart disease.

All in all, choosing an all-natural plant-based diet can have an incredible impact on your health and help prevent and arrest chronic degenerative diseases. See Chapter 2 for more on this.

Eating Meat Impacts Climate Change

The impact that meat consumption continues to have on climate change is quite intense. Although most people wouldn't associate the two, here's a bit of the picture: To keep up with the demand for meat, cows are fed an incredible amount of food, which produces waste. This waste gives off methane gases, which contribute to ozone depletion by trapping heat in the atmosphere. Take the number of feedlots that exist across the world and multiply that by the amount of waste made each day by farm animals, and you've got a lot of gases making the world a scarier place by the minute. In addition, enormous amounts of carbon dioxide stored in trees are released during the destruction of vast acres of forest to provide pastureland and to grow crops for farmed animals.

Additionally, manufacturing one calorie from animal protein requires 11 times as much fossil fuel input as producing a calorie from plant protein. Why is this bad? Burning fossil fuels (such as oil and gasoline) releases carbon dioxide, the primary gas responsible for climate change.

By choosing to eat more plants over meat, you're choosing to not contribute to this vicious cycle. Not only that, the more plants are farmed, the more beneficial gases (such as oxygen) are produced for the atmosphere.

Eating Meat Is Cruel

As a result of the increase in demand for meat, factory farms (large, industrialized farms on which large numbers of livestock are raised indoors in conditions intended to maximize production at minimal cost) are on the rise.

What this means is that animals are treated with no respect. How would you feel being crowded into a small space, with no room to run around, lift your hand, or even sit down? This is truly the case for most animals these days, and it's all for the purpose of fast, cheap, money-making production. Very little care is taken for the animals' welfare. They're given antibiotics to combat the infections they get from living in such close quarters and growth hormones to increase their size and weight in an unnaturally short period of time (and both of these things eventually wind up in your food).

An old saying goes, "If slaughterhouses had glass walls, everyone would be vegetarian." You can find many ways to inform yourself about some of these actions; check out resources such as documentaries, books, and websites. These are some of my favorites:

- **Documentaries:** *Earthlings; Death on a Factory Farm: Food, Inc.; Vegucated; Forks over Knives;* and *Food Matters*

- **Websites:** www.peta.org, www.meat.org, www.farmsanctuary. org, www.themeatrix.com, www.humanesociety.org, and www. nutritionfacts.org

- **Books:** *That's Why We Don't Eat Animals* by Ruby Roth (North Atlantic Books), *Eating Animals* by Jonathan Safran Foer (Back Bay Books), *The China Study* by T. Colin Campbell and Thomas M. Campbell II (BenBella Books), and *Whole: Rethinking the Science of Nutrition* by T. Colin Campbell (BenBella Books)

The Meat Industry Is Getting Worse

The more control mankind has had over food, the worse it has gotten. This is apparent with packaged foods but especially with animal-based foods. Obviously, an increased demand for meat has strained the supply chain. To put enough meat on the shelves at inexpensive prices, farmers have put into place often-unsustainable practices. This can mean manipulating the environments in which animals are raised, which can lead to contamination of the animal feed, the soil, the land, and ultimately the meat on your plate. It's no wonder that every couple of years we hear about some bacteria, such as salmonella or E. coli, that has found its way into our food.

Here are just a few more things happening in the animal industry that affect not only animals' lives but ours, as well.

- Contamination of animal feed ultimately infects our food supply with superbugs, E. coli, and mad-cow disease.

- Farmers are using more growth hormones to raise animals.

- Organic farming practices are underused because they aren't as economically efficient.

Index

• D •

• *E* •

• I •

• J •

• K •

About the Author

Simply said, Marni Wasserman's life is rooted in healthy eating. As a culinary nutritionist, health strategist, and owner of Toronto's first plant-based food studio, Marni uses passion and experience to educate individuals on how to adopt a realistic plant-based diet that is both simple and delicious. She is dedicated to providing individuals with balanced, nutritious choices through organic, fresh, whole, and natural plant-based foods and other natural lifestyle modalities.

Marni is a graduate of the Institute of Holistic Nutrition in Toronto (where she is now on the faculty) and the Natural Gourmet Culinary School in New York, and she is the founder of Marni Wasserman's Food Studio & Lifestyle Shop in Midtown Toronto. This is where she teaches her signature cooking classes and offers collaborative workshops and urban retreats. Her food studio is also a place where people can purchase sustainable superfoods and lifestyle products. It was recognized as one of Toronto's top ten cooking schools in 2008.

As a prominent expert on health and nutrition, Marni writes a column called "Nourish" in *Tonic Toronto* magazine. She is also a contributor to the *Huffington Post* and *Chatelaine Magazine* and has made several TV appearances. She's consulted with one of Toronto's prominent hotels — the Windsor Arms Hotel — for vegan and vegetarian menus and participates in several speaking and cooking demonstrations throughout the year.

Marni is also the co-author of *Fermenting For Dummies* and several well-received e-books.

You can learn more about Marni by visiting her on Facebook (`marnisfood studio`), following her on Twitter (`@marniwasserman`), checking out her Pinterest page (`www.pinterest.com/fullynourished`), or visiting her website (`www.marniwasserman.com`).

Dedication

This book is dedicated to anyone who wants to adopt a healthier way of eating and living. This book is also for all those people who are looking to support and inspire themselves, friends, or family members to take on a plant-based diet.

Author's Acknowledgments

I would like to express thanks to the team at Wiley for asking me to be the author of *Plant-Based Diet For Dummies*. The core team with which I've been working closely to make this book come to life includes Sarah Sypniewski, Dummifier; Vicki Adang, senior project editor; and Tracy Boggier, senior acquisitions editor. You have helped keep me going at every step along the way. In addition, I would like to acknowledge Ashley Petry, copy editor; Emily Nolan, recipe tester; and Tracey Eakin, technical editor, for making sure everything I wrote makes sense and looks and tastes good!

Publisher's Acknowledgments

Contributor: Sarah Sypniewski

Senior Acquisitions Editor: Tracy Boggier

Senior Project Editor: Victoria M. Adang

Copy Editor: Ashley Petry

Technical Editor: Tracey A. Eakin
(www.traceyeakin.com)

Art Coordinator: Alicia B. South

Project Coordinator: Lauren Buroker

Illustrator: Elizabeth Kurtzman

Cover Image: © iStockphoto.com/Albuquerque

Apple & Mac

iPad For Dummies,
5th Edition
978-1-118-72306-7

iPhone For Dummies,
7th Edition
978-1-118-69083-3

Macs All-in-One
For Dummies, 4th Edition
978-1-118-82210-4

OS X Mavericks
For Dummies
978-1-118-69188-5

Blogging & Social Media

Facebook For Dummies,
5th Edition
978-1-118-63312-0

Social Media Engagement
For Dummies
978-1-118-53019-1

WordPress For Dummies,
6th Edition
978-1-118-79161-5

Business

Stock Investing
For Dummies, 4th Edition
978-1-118-37678-2

Investing For Dummies,
6th Edition
978-0-470-90545-6

Personal Finance
For Dummies, 7th Edition
978-1-118-11785-9

QuickBooks 2014
For Dummies
978-1-118-72005-9

Small Business Marketing
Kit For Dummies,
3rd Edition
978-1-118-31183-7

Careers

Job Interviews
For Dummies, 4th Edition
978-1-118-11290-8

Job Searching with Social
Media For Dummies,
2nd Edition
978-1-118-67856-5

Personal Branding
For Dummies
978-1-118-11792-7

Resumes For Dummies,
6th Edition
978-0-470-87361-8

Starting an Etsy Business
For Dummies, 2nd Edition
978-1-118-59024-9

Diet & Nutrition

Belly Fat Diet For Dummies
978-1-118-34585-6

Mediterranean Diet
For Dummies
978-1-118-71525-3

Nutrition For Dummies,
5th Edition
978-0-470-93231-5

Digital Photography

Digital SLR Photography
All-in-One For Dummies,
2nd Edition
978-1-118-59082-9

Digital SLR Video &
Filmmaking For Dummies
978-1-118-36598-4

Photoshop Elements 12
For Dummies
978-1-118-72714-0

Gardening

Herb Gardening
For Dummies, 2nd Edition
978-0-470-61778-6

Gardening with Free-Range
Chickens For Dummies
978-1-118-54754-0

Health

Boosting Your Immunity
For Dummies
978-1-118-40200-9

Diabetes For Dummies,
4th Edition
978-1-118-29447-5

Living Paleo For Dummies
978-1-118-29405-5

Big Data

Big Data For Dummies
978-1-118-50422-2

Data Visualization
For Dummies
978-1-118-50289-1

Hadoop For Dummies
978-1-118-60755-8

Language &
Foreign Language

500 Spanish Verbs
For Dummies
978-1-118-02382-2

English Grammar
For Dummies, 2nd Edition
978-0-470-54664-2

French All-in-One
For Dummies
978-1-118-22815-9

German Essentials
For Dummies
978-1-118-18422-6

Italian For Dummies,
2nd Edition
978-1-118-00465-4

Available in print and e-book formats.

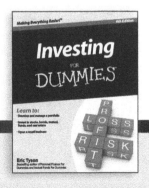
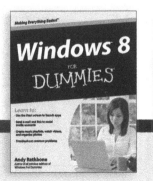
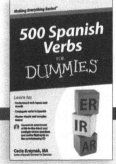
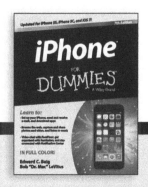

Available wherever books are sold. **For more information or to order direct visit www.dummies.com**

Math & Science

Algebra I For Dummies, 2nd Edition
978-0-470-55964-2

Anatomy and Physiology For Dummies, 2nd Edition
978-0-470-92326-9

Astronomy For Dummies, 3rd Edition
978-1-118-37697-3

Biology For Dummies, 2nd Edition
978-0-470-59875-7

Chemistry For Dummies, 2nd Edition
978-1-118-00730-3

1001 Algebra II Practice Problems For Dummies
978-1-118-44662-1

Microsoft Office

Excel 2013 For Dummies
978-1-118-51012-4

Office 2013 All-in-One For Dummies
978-1-118-51636-2

PowerPoint 2013 For Dummies
978-1-118-50253-2

Word 2013 For Dummies
978-1-118-49123-2

Music

Blues Harmonica For Dummies
978-1-118-25269-7

Guitar For Dummies, 3rd Edition
978-1-118-11554-1

iPod & iTunes For Dummies, 10th Edition
978-1-118-50864-0

Programming

Beginning Programming with C For Dummies
978-1-118-73763-7

Excel VBA Programming For Dummies, 3rd Edition
978-1-118-49037-2

Java For Dummies, 6th Edition
978-1-118-40780-6

Religion & Inspiration

The Bible For Dummies
978-0-7645-5296-0

Buddhism For Dummies, 2nd Edition
978-1-118-02379-2

Catholicism For Dummies, 2nd Edition
978-1-118-07778-8

Self-Help & Relationships

Beating Sugar Addiction For Dummies
978-1-118-54645-1

Meditation For Dummies, 3rd Edition
978-1-118-29144-3

Seniors

Laptops For Seniors For Dummies, 3rd Edition
978-1-118-71105-7

Computers For Seniors For Dummies, 3rd Edition
978-1-118-11553-4

iPad For Seniors For Dummies, 6th Edition
978-1-118-72826-0

Social Security For Dummies
978-1-118-20573-0

Smartphones & Tablets

Android Phones For Dummies, 2nd Edition
978-1-118-72030-1

Nexus Tablets For Dummies
978-1-118-77243-0

Samsung Galaxy S 4 For Dummies
978-1-118-64222-1

Samsung Galaxy Tabs For Dummies
978-1-118-77294-2

Test Prep

ACT For Dummies, 5th Edition
978-1-118-01259-8

ASVAB For Dummies, 3rd Edition
978-0-470-63760-9

GRE For Dummies, 7th Edition
978-0-470-88921-3

Officer Candidate Tests For Dummies
978-0-470-59876-4

Physician's Assistant Exam For Dummies
978-1-118-11556-5

Series 7 Exam For Dummie
978-0-470-09932-2

Windows 8

Windows 8.1 All-in-One For Dummies
978-1-118-82087-2

Windows 8.1 For Dummies
978-1-118-82121-3

Windows 8.1 For Dummies Book + DVD Bundle
978-1-118-82107-7

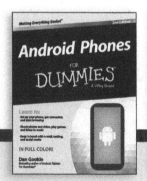 **Available in print and e-book formats.**

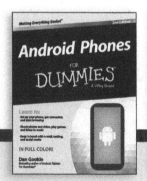 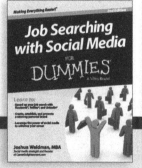 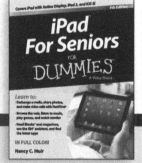 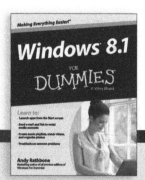

Take Dummies with you everywhere you go!

Whether you are excited about e-books, want more from the web, must have your mobile apps, or are swept up in social media, Dummies makes everything easier.

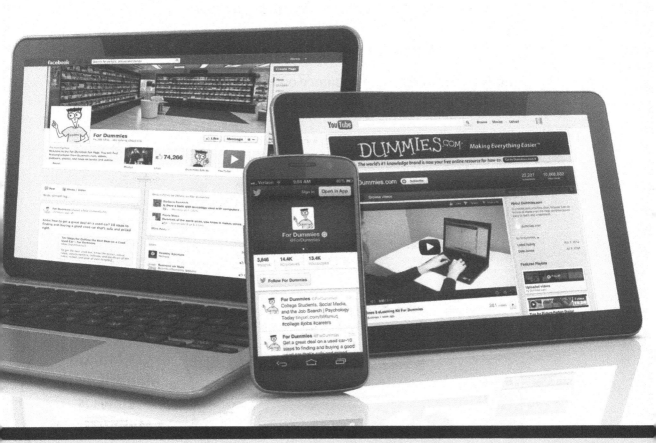

Leverage the Power

For Dummies is the global leader in the reference category and one of the most trusted and highly regarded brands in the world. No longer just focused on books, customers now have access to the For Dummies content they need in the format they want. Let us help you develop a solution that will fit your brand and help you connect with your customers.

Advertising & Sponsorships

Connect with an engaged audience on a powerful multimedia site, and position your message alongside expert how-to content.

Targeted ads • Video • Email marketing • Microsites • Sweepstakes sponsorship

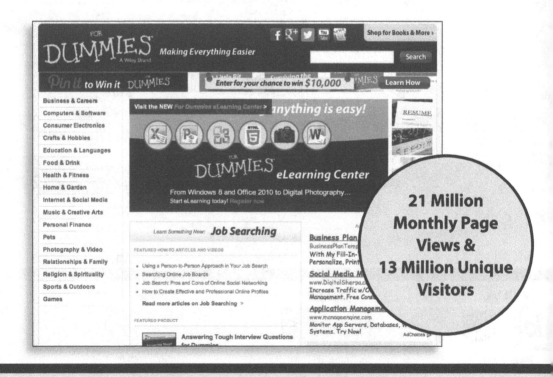

21 Million Monthly Page Views & 13 Million Unique Visitors